I0753586

GOD SAID

a personal testament of hope by KAT FLIPPIN

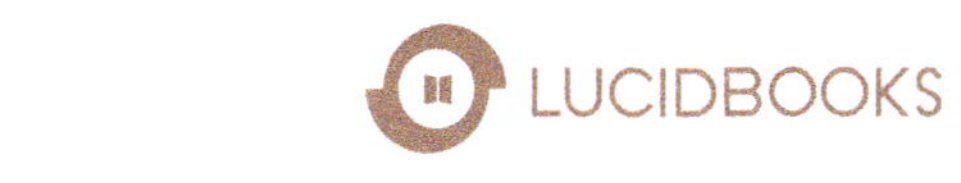

God Said: A Personal Testament of Hope

Cover design and art by The Branding Co.
Photography by Ashley Dankert Photography

Published by Lucid Books in Houston, TX
www.LucidBooks.com

Emphasis in Scripture shown by italics, bold, or underline are the author's.

ISBN: 978-1-63296-692-6
eISBN: 978-1-63296-693-3

Special Sales: Most Lucid Books titles are available in special quantity discounts. Custom imprinting or excerpting can also be done to fit special needs. Contact Lucid Books at Info@LucidBooks.com

Content

i. | Preface

Preface

Something that you'll learn about me is that I have an image of an olive branch or olive tree on almost all my social media profile pages, in my office, on my computer wallpaper, and my cell phone wallpaper. If you ask me why olive trees carry so much significance in my life, you may want to grab a cup of coffee or tea and make yourself comfortable. You're in for quite a story.

- The olive tree is one of the most resilient trees on the planet. It survived the worldwide flood described in Genesis 7:1–9:17. According to the Olive Grove Oundle web page, olive trees are known to not only survive but thrive during seasons of drought, sub-zero temperatures, frost, and even fire.[1]

- The oldest olive trees are estimated to be around 2,000 years old! Olive trees can even bear fruit at over 1,000 years old. Incredible!

- Olive tree roots are so strong that they can re-grow even when the tree itself has been decimated. If the roots are intact, the olive tree can rise above the soil again. Shoots can even grow from an olive tree stump and continue to bear fruit again.

- The olive tree and olives carry so much correlation to Jesus. When the olives are collected at harvest, the first thing that is done is that they are crushed. *"But he was pierced for our transgressions, he was crushed for our iniquities; the punishment that brought us peace was on him, and by his wounds we are healed."* (Isaiah 53:5 NIV)

- Olives are crushed into a paste and put into a basket. Then twelve baskets are piled up on top of each other and pressed for hours.

- To produce oil, olives are pressed three times. Olive oil produced from the *first pressing*, "first oil," is what we know as "extra virgin oil." This was the oil used to light the menorah and anoint kings, priests, and prophets. The oil from the *second pressing* is used for perfume, cosmetics, cooking, and medicinal purposes. The oil from the third pressing is used for candles and soap. When Jesus was crucified on the cross, his "pressing" resulted in our anointing, healing through His blood, and cleansing from sins (salvation).

- During The Flood, olive trees were underwater for over a year and not destroyed. When the waters receded, it was an olive branch that the dove brought back to Noah. While the olive branch symbolizes peace, what that means to me personally is that floods of grief, loss, or pain may come against me in this life, but I have the peace of Jesus thriving inside. I am planted or rooted in Him. I cannot be moved or destroyed.

- To me, the olive tree and the olive represent new life, abundance, glory, resilience, and strength. "Your wife will be like a fruitful grapevine, flourishing within your home. Your children will be like vigorous young olive trees as they sit around your table." (Psalm 128:3)

- After experiencing seven miscarriages, I look at the olive tree as a symbol of what I carry inside. With every loss, I dug my roots deeper and deeper into Jesus as my source of peace and strength. His faithful promises bore new life and shoots from where I felt cut down to a stump.

That's why I see unshakable beauty and value in the olive tree and all that it represents.

ii. | Introduction

Introduction

THERE IS SOMETHING VERY POWERFUL ABOUT THE SPOKEN WORD. One word of encouragement can make someone feel empowered and unstoppable. While one word of accusation, rejection, or discouragement can make someone quit or even believe a lie about their identity—about who they really are. The impact of words is huge. The words that come out of our mouths bring life or death. *"Death and life are in the power of the tongue."* (Proverbs 18:21a NASB2020) We build people up or we tear them down; this also applies to our self-talk. What we speak over ourselves impacts what we believe and the choices that direct our lives and our futures.

This book is my heart on paper. I'm stepping out in vulnerability to share my story of repeated miscarriages, my struggles through grief and despair, what the healing process looked like for me, and what God can do with pain on the other side of it all. My prayer is that this story will bring you hope and instill in you the courage to trust God through your own healing process. You may discover a new way to encounter God in the midst of whatever you are facing right now. Grief and loss can feel incredibly heavy. My hope is that these words will inspire and motivate you toward that next step to healing and freedom. Know that you are not alone in your pain.

In full disclosure, this book will be a very raw read. You will be walking through my story, the healing process, and the revelations discovered through it all. I share candid journal entries that describe my experiences, thoughts, and emotions as they were occurring in real time. You'll get to see my candid conversations with God and my thoughts as I wrestled with the injustices that life was handing me.

At the end of each chapter, I included lifelines (Scripture verses, songs, quotes, and sermons) that got me through my toughest moments. Feel free to choose the verses, songs, quotes, sermons, and so on that speak the most to your heart and hold them close. I also included a resource library at the end of the book with links to my video testimony and worship playlists, which you can access at any time. Everyone's story looks different, but maybe my story can provide some hope and draw you closer to God as you walk through yours.

I was absolutely terrified of healing. I was convinced that having to relive my pain and deepest wounds would make healing the hardest and most painful process. Picture a dam built stone by stone holding back a reservoir of pain and anguish. That was what I had done internally with the pain I was carrying. Every stone represented a moment when I chose to stop feeling and push the pain back. With a dam of emotions being carefully held back, the mere suggestion of going through the healing process put my precarious compartmentalization in danger. I honestly believed that if I started to dismantle that carefully constructed wall of pain, I would be crushed by the stones, and then drown in despair. But relationship with God is surprising—it has a way of breathing life over death. Light breaks through darkness. In the middle of the worst of it, I found that I was not alone and that if I allowed Him to come along with me through the process and carry the pain, I could experience freedom, joy, peace, and a lightness in my spirit. Yes, the things we read in Scripture are real and do apply to us.

> *For all that I require of you will be pleasant and easy to bear.*
>
> – Matthew 11:30 TPT

> *The LORD is close to the brokenhearted; He rescues those whose spirits are crushed.*
>
> – Psalm 34:18

> *He will wipe every tear from their eyes, and there will be no more death or sorrow or crying or pain. All these things are gone forever.*
>
> – Revelation 21:4

The word of God has made the most significant impact on my life. The Bible has hundreds of stories bearing witness to God's faithfulness, answered prayers, fulfilled promises, impossible miracles, and deliverance. The Israelites got to see with their own eyes God empowering Moses to part the Red Sea so that nearly 2 million Israelites could walk through to freedom on dry ground. Sarah became pregnant at ninety years old. Jericho's walls fell after the Israelites simply walked around the city in circles and then shouted with praise. What?! The Bible is full of amazing stories in which God heard the cries of His people and did the impossible. I grew up in church and heard many of those stories over and over again. But they were just stories until it got personal. God broke through my darkness and did the impossible in my life. I now know without a doubt that when God speaks a single word, it is done.

If you hear me say anything in this book, hear loud and clear that you and I have an Almighty, living God who can break through the darkest of nights and bring hope where it seems impossible. God loves us, advocates for us, and fights for us more than we know. He doesn't reach down into our pit from a distance to pull us out; instead, He climbs down into our pit and walks out with us. God can be trusted to keep His promises. He is a God who restores what has been lost, and He is faithful!

But before I get too far ahead of myself, you should know that I was scared to death to share my story. The Holy Spirit whispered in my ear, "Write a book. Share your story." I smiled and thought, "That's nice. Um... I've never written a book. How am I supposed to do this? I'm just a regular person." Plenty of books concerning grief and hope have been written by pillars in the Christian community. Pastor Craig Groeschel wrote *Hope in the Dark*, Bishop T. D. Jakes wrote *Crushing*, Beth Moore wrote *Get Out of That Pit*, and Lysa TerKeurst wrote *It's not Supposed to Be This Way* to name just a few. You get the idea. If I share my story, I reasoned, it might be a super-depressing read. Who wants to read about grief? Nope. We have enough sadness in this life. Why read about it too? You can clearly see how this conversation with the Holy Spirit was going. Take note of how easy it is to talk yourself out of your calling.

Then a good friend was visiting one day, and we had an opportunity to read through a couple of journal entries I had written. Ironically, I was sharing those journal entries in an effort to offer encouragement and hope despite what I just said about my story being a depressing read. My friend called me out on the spot and said, "You are a writer, and God already told you to start writing a book, hasn't He?" Sigh. I got outed by God. "Yes, He has." There was no hiding from it now. I immediately tried to make an excuse about my abilities as a writer or lack thereof; however, my words betrayed me as we surveyed the stack of seven journals filled with all my conversations with God regarding pain, hope, desperate prayers, and triumphs dating back almost twenty years. Yep, no denying it now. I owned it and confessed for the first time out loud.

I'm a writer.

I definitely had moments when the thought of writing a book seemed daunting and I felt incredibly vulnerable. What would people think? How would my words be received? But if God asked me to do it, then my only responsibility was to be obedient, share my story, and let God do the rest. Anytime that there was a lull in the progress of writing this book, God would chase me down and even send strangers to tell me, "You're a writer, aren't you?" And then I'd instantly be reminded how urgent and important it was to share my story with others.

It is my heart's longing that as we go through these pages together, you will be emboldened to take a first step of courage toward inviting God into your story. You are not alone, and God can be trusted to keep His word. I challenge you to hold God to His word. You won't be disappointed. Let me show you what I mean.

> Heavenly Father, I ask that Your words come through these pages. Use this story for Your glory. I ask for breakthroughs and that we will experience

You in a new way. Allow us to feel Your presence and to understand that You are a safe place. You can be trusted. Please protect our hearts and guard our minds against the lies that try to take control. Help us to surrender and experience Your rest and peace and freedom. Thank You for being so faithful and true to Your word. In Jesus' name, Amen.

part 1 | *The Journey*

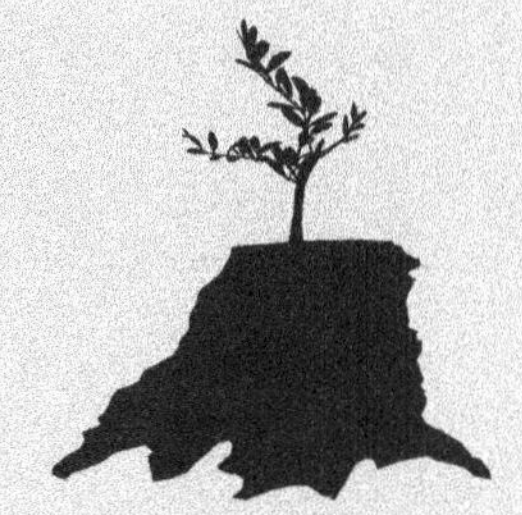

GOD SAID... *hold on to hope.*

Hope

But blessed are those who trust in the LORD and have made the LORD their hope and confidence. –Jeremiah 17:7

PREGNANCY IS SUCH A WONDER. You feel joyous, empowered, and utterly helpless all at once. What a miracle it is to be growing a baby. A fertilized egg starts to develop, and those little cells multiply over and over again. Growth is rapid and at just five weeks into the process, the heart starts to beat. I'm in awe at the process in which all this rapid growth—blood flow, formation of the heart and vital organs—is sustained in the beginning stages by the hormones released from the ovary. When I learned this, I was incredibly surprised! I previously thought that the umbilical cord sustained and nurtured the baby from the beginning through delivery, but the umbilical cord doesn't come into play until about ten to twelve weeks into the pregnancy. Truly miraculous!!

The honor of motherhood is birthed with that first positive pregnancy test. Motherhood. Wow. What a huge and humbling honor. My first step into motherhood started in 2006. My husband and I were two years into married life when we received the happy news that our sweet little one was on the way. With the news of the pregnancy, we, of course, told everyone. We were so excited! We started picking out names and planning all the details of the nursery. Our world had just exploded with hope and joy and possibility.

There is nothing like the hope of a first baby.

> Journal Entries from February 7 and 8, 2006:
>
> Good morning, Lord. I'm sorry it's been a while since I've spent some real quality time with You. Flip and I found out last Thursday, February 2nd,

that we're going to have a baby. Thank you for all your blessings! We are so excited! We are most likely going to wait until the baby is born to find out if it's a boy or a girl. Flip wants it to be a surprise. I still can't believe we're going to have a baby. My first doctor's appointment is on March 1st at eight thirty in the morning. I'm nervous and excited at the same time! I'm definitely being made aware of all of the changes going on with my body. My emotions are like a roller coaster. I'm happy and perfectly fine one moment, and then I'm crying and frustrated at everything. I actually annoy myself. I keep apologizing to Flip and thanking him for being such a wonderful husband.

Journal Entry from March 8, 2006:

I had my first doctor's appointment last Wednesday. It was mostly just a checkup for me. The nurse practitioner tried to listen for a heartbeat, but she couldn't hear anything. Lori (Flip's mom) left a doppler at our house so we can try to hear for it ourselves. It should be soon. My next appointment is on March 16 in Roseville. Lori and my mom are going to try to come so they can push for an ultrasound. We all want to know if I have twins. It's all very exciting!

God, thank You for the blessing of having a baby. We look forward to all the miraculous ways You will provide for our little family. We look forward to all the lessons You will teach us through our baby. Thank You for the blessing.

A first baby is precious. Never once did we ever consider that it could all disappear.

Journal Entry from March 20, 2006:

Hi. The last week has been very painful. Our little baby is no longer alive. The doctor couldn't hear a heartbeat, so she did an ultrasound. There was no heartbeat. She said that our baby probably stopped growing/living at about ten weeks old. There was no explanation. The doctor reassured us over and over again that we did nothing wrong. It's very devastating. My heart is broken. Flip cried in my lap at the doctor's office.

We don't understand, and we cry frequently. This coming Thursday I go in for surgery to have our little one removed. The doctor said there would be too much blood and possible infection for me to pass our baby naturally. Thursday will be a sad day.

> *When doubts filled my mind, your comfort gave me renewed hope and cheer.*
>
> – Psalm 94:19
>
> *Your promise revives me; it comforts me in all my troubles.*
>
> – Psalm 119:50
>
> *So we have been greatly encouraged in the midst of our troubles and suffering, dear brothers and sisters, because you have remained strong in your faith.*
>
> – 1 Thessalonians 3:7
>
> *May integrity and honesty protect me, for I put my hope in You.*
>
> – Psalm 25:21
>
> *O LORD, you alone are my hope. I've trusted you, O LORD, from childhood.*
>
> – Psalm 71:5
>
> *I pray that God, the source of hope, will fill you completely with joy and peace because you trust in him. Then you will overflow with confident hope through the power of the Holy Spirit.*
>
> – Romans 15:13

> Journal Entry from March 22, 2006:
>
> Good morning, Lord. I am somewhat numb. I want to cry, but I seem to be out of tears. My heart is grieving, but I almost act as if I was never pregnant. I don't know how to feel. God, please comfort me. Wrap Your arms around me and don't let go. My heart is sad. My baby leaves my body tomorrow. Help me.

The only way to describe it is like being gutted. The doctor told us that the baby had stopped growing around ten weeks and that because my body wasn't naturally miscarrying, we needed to schedule a D&C. I wasn't sure what a D&C was. For those who don't know:

> A dilation and curettage procedure, also called a D&C, is a surgical procedure in which the cervix (lower, narrow part of the uterus) is dilated (expanded) so that the uterine lining (endometrium) can be scraped with a curette (spoon-shaped instrument) to remove abnormal tissues.[2]

Even worse than preparing to be physically gutted was the waiting. The D&C

couldn't be scheduled for two weeks, so I continued to carry our deceased child until it was time. When I arrived at the clinic, everyone was there for the same thing. It was a quick outpatient 20-minute procedure. I felt like livestock being processed. After the procedure, I woke up in a room full of beds with other recovering girls and women. You could hear whimpering echo throughout the recovery room. The atmosphere was full of anguish, pain, grief, and hopelessness. In a word, I felt "empty."

I remember watching my husband cry in the doctor's office. It's a rare event to see my husband cry, and that memory will always be with me. I remember retracing everything I ate and wondered if I could've changed the outcome. Did I drink coffee? Did I take a shower that was too hot? Did I exercise too aggressively? Did my heart rate get too high? What could I have done differently? How could I have spared my sweet baby? What do you do when there are no answers? You might think the natural response would be to blame God. I thought about it, but I mostly blamed myself. It was easy to blame myself. I was the one who was pregnant.

It's shocking how many people don't know how to respond to grief, particularly within the church. I had an expectation that other believers would somehow provide solace or comfort or maybe even have answers to help me reconcile our loss. But what I found were people who (1) didn't know what to say, (2) encouraged us to move on, or (3) offered advice on how to succeed with a healthy pregnancy in the future. In trying to put myself in their shoes, I admit that it is awkward to know what to say. When great loss occurs, there is a permanence to it that words cannot console. How do you make someone feel better? You can't. You kinda need to just sit in their pain with them and allow them to process in their own time.

We had well-meaning people tell us, "Don't worry. You're young. You have plenty of time to have more babies." "Miscarriages are common." "Your body is warmed up now. Getting pregnant again shouldn't be a problem." These words were no comfort to us. We were not ready to hope for another baby. We wanted the one we lost.

I also learned the harsh reality that life doesn't stop when you feel like your heart has. Culture doesn't seem to allow the space and time to fully grieve when loss occurs. You might be able to take a few days off work, but physical and emotional healing needs more time. With the shortage of time to grieve, life requires you to shove the pain down, put on a brave face, and return to household demands, work obligations, and church expectations. Act like nothing happened.

Emotionally, I built a layer around my heart to protect myself. I shoved the pain down, distracted myself, and carried on.

> I've learned that grieving is not the time to look for answers; it takes all your energy just to survive the turbulence of the loss. And truth be told, there is no philosophical or theological comprehension that can adequately articulate the pain radiating from one whose soul cries out in silent sorrow.
> – Bishop T. D. Jakes[3]

While my heart was still raw, a dear friend reached out to me and shared that she too had experienced the loss of a baby. She handed me a gift. It was a Willow Tree figurine of a child holding a wire balloon with the word HOPE inside it. She told me to disregard all the foolish things that others might say in their attempts to comfort and to celebrate the fact that I am a mother and carried life inside me, even if only for a short while. She said that it helps to have something physical to hold and remember. I was incredibly grateful for her kindness and for the words of life she spoke over me when I was feeling such loss. And she's right. I greatly treasured that little Willow Tree figurine with the word HOPE. I have it to this day.

> *Gentle words are a tree of life.*
>
> – Proverbs 15:4a

> *Kind words are like honey—sweet to the soul and healthy for the body.*
> – Proverbs 16:24

Journal Entry from March 28, 2006:

This month has been a month of disappointment, heartache, grief, sadness, dashed hopes, and fears coming true. I feel that You are preparing us for something great, but the process hurts. My heart is in pain. I am afraid to hope. Please help me, comfort me, hold me. Teach me how to put my hope in You and not my circumstances. I am afraid.

> *I prayed to the LORD, and he answered me, freeing me from all my fears.*
>
> – Psalm 34:4

> *Do not fear anything except the Lord Almighty. He alone is the Holy One. If you fear Him, you need fear nothing else.*
>
> – Isaiah 8:13

God, why am I so scared? I trust You and that You will take care of us and guide us. But I know that Your will be done no matter what and I don't want to hurt anymore. I'm scared that the next step in our lives will produce more pain and heartache. Is there such a thing as a season of prosperity and joy? Is that an unattainable dream in this life? Please grant me something to hope for.

> *We can make our plans, but the LORD determines our steps.*
>
> – Proverbs 16:9

Lifelines

QUESTIONS TO CONSIDER

When grief and loss strike unexpectedly, how do you respond? Do you typically respond with anger, blame, withdrawal, or numbness?

Are you able to trust God with your pain? Tell Him how you feel.

SCRIPTURE VERSES

“For I know the plans I have for you,” says the LORD. “They are plans for good and not for disaster, to give you a future and a hope.” –Jeremiah 29:11

When doubts filled my mind, your comfort gave me renewed hope and cheer. – Psalms 94:19

Your promise revives me; it comforts me in all my troubles. – Psalms 119:50

So we have been greatly comforted, dear brothers and sisters, in all of our own crushing troubles and suffering, because you have remained strong in your faith. – I Thessalonians 3:7

WORSHIP SONGS

"Even When It Hurts (Praise Song)" by Hillsong UNITED from the *Of Dirt and Grace (Live from the Land)* album.

"Needing You Now" by Meredith Andrews and We Are Messengers from the *My Utmost For His Highest* album.

"Rescue" by Lauren Daigle from her *Look Up Child* album.

QUOTES

"May your choices reflect your hopes, not your fears." - Nelson Mandela[4]

"I've learned that grieving is not the time to look for answers; it takes all your energy just to survive the turbulence of the loss. And truth be told, there is no philosophical or theological comprehension that can adequately articulate the pain radiating from one whose soul cries out in silent sorrow."
- Bishop T.D. Jakes[5]

PRAYER

God, I ask for Your peace and comfort to surround us in the middle of our current season of deep loss and grief. The pain feels like a gut punch and can take our breath away, but God, remind us of Your presence and that You haven't left us even for a second. Allow us to feel Your love and speak hope into our hearts right now. In Jesus' powerful name, Amen.

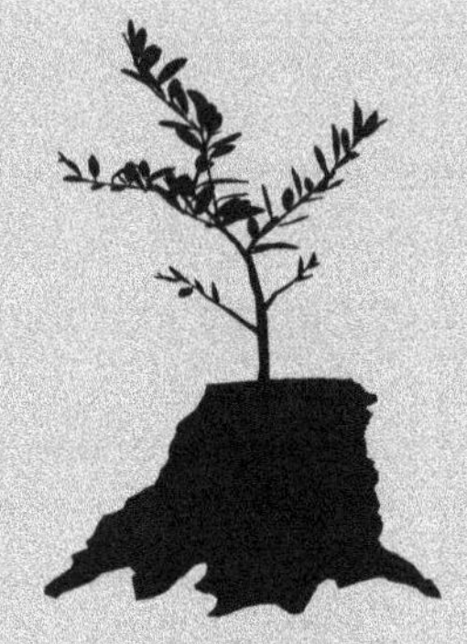

GOD SAID... *have faith.*

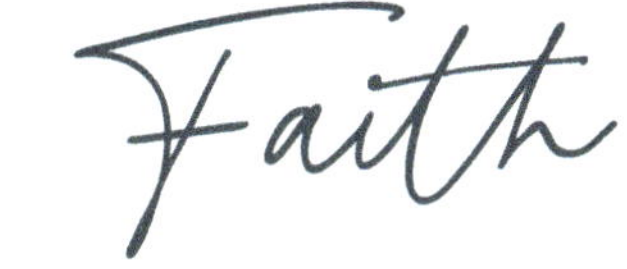

Faith shows the reality of what we hope for; it is the evidence of things we cannot yet see. – Hebrews 11:1

SHEER JOY AND PARALYZING FEAR in one confusing, complicated package. I was twenty-three years old when we were pregnant with our first. It was a surprise to us because we weren't trying to get pregnant at the time. The comfort of time provided us the courage to try again. Five years passed before we found out that we were pregnant again. You might think that those five years provided us with time to heal from our loss, but we stayed really busy running a youth group and working sixty hours per week and didn't allow ourselves to think about the loss. With the news of this second pregnancy, we were very excited, but also keenly reminded about the potential of losing this one as well. We didn't have any answers as to what caused the first loss, so we stepped into this second pregnancy with a lot of unknowns.

> Journal Entry from September 28, 2010:
>
> The biggest surprise of last week is that we learned on September 23rd that we are pregnant! It was quite a shock, and we were filled with excitement and fear all at the same moment. We are understandably nervous and anxiously waiting to hear that little heartbeat with our own ears. We are waiting to tell anyone until we hear the heartbeat, and then we can start making announcements.
>
> *Yes, give praise, O servants of the LORD. Praise the name of the LORD! Blessed be the name of the LORD forever and ever... He gives the barren woman a home, so that she becomes a happy mother. Praise the LORD!*
>
> – Psalm 113:1–2, 9

We went to the doctor seven weeks into the pregnancy, and our fears came rushing right back into reality again. The news was not good. The doctor let us know that there was no heartbeat, and that this pregnancy was not viable. I had grown to despise the phrase "not viable." It's cold, and I felt so empty and broken.

We were provided with instructions to prepare for another D&C. The morning of the procedure, I ended up miscarrying naturally in the shower. While it felt like my heart was bleeding right along with my body, something very special happened with this sweet baby that I have not experienced again. When I lost this one, I was able to hold our newly formed baby in my hands. The baby was the size of my pinky finger, and I could see a little head and hands and feet. For a brief moment, I got a glimpse at the miracle of life, and it was beautiful. It also made me aware of how many things have to go perfectly right for life to happen. In Psalm 139:14, David is not exaggerating when he says how fearfully and wonderfully we are made.

> Journal Entry from November 19, 2010:
>
> God, I have finally found some quiet time to spend alone with You. I'm sorry I have been keeping You at arm's length. I know how well You know me, and I was afraid to confront the pain in my life right now.
>
> We have lost another baby, and the pain was almost too much to bear. It is amazing to think we have come through this with a determined hope to try again. This time was so different from the last. We were surrounded with good friends and encouragement from church. We were so blessed. Our home was bright with bouquets of flowers for about two weeks.
>
> Mom also came for a few days to offer support and a shoulder to cry on. We were scheduled for a D&C and ended up miscarrying the morning of the surgery. Our little unborn life fell out while I was in the shower. I will never forget the image of that little life.

> Journal Entry from November 20, 2010:
>
> *When you go through deep waters, I will be with you. When you go through rivers of difficulty, you will not drown. When you walk through the fire of oppression, you will not be burned up; the flames will not consume you. For I am the LORD, your God, the Holy One of Israel, your Savior. I gave Egypt as a ransom for your freedom; I gave Ethiopia and Seba in your place.*
>
> *– Isaiah 43:2–3*

> I absolutely love that this passage says "When" and not "If." Great trouble, difficulty, and oppression will happen, but my God is greater, my God is stronger, my God is higher than any other. Nothing can touch me. God promises to always be with me. I will not drown or be consumed.

When any loss is experienced, it feels like a great injustice has occurred. Life doesn't ask for your permission. It's harsh and unapologetic. Having experienced this second loss brought with it a sense of permanence, making it more challenging to hope for a different outcome in the future. A week after our sad news, some very dear friends of ours came over to our apartment with dinner. No words needed to be spoken. They sat with us on the couch. We ate food and binge-watched Chopped on the Food Network. It allowed us to be distracted from the heartache for a bit. Their simply being present with us was more healing than anything we even knew to ask for at the time. When pain is overwhelming, distraction is a blessing to the mind.

Looking back on it now, I can see how I had to force myself to take a deep breath and shove the pain down again. I didn't know what to do with it. There was no way I was going to unleash this anguish on an unsuspecting friend.

Eight months passed, and I was still wrestling with hope. Was it even possible to continue to hope?

> Journal Entry from July 12, 2011:
>
> For the first time in years, God has somehow arranged a date with me. My alarm went off an hour early, and I find myself with extra time before work. Flip urged me to spend the time journaling. He's a wise man.
>
> So here I am sitting at the park. The flowers are in bloom; there are vines growing up all around this table; it's green, cool, and beautiful. God, thank You for where we live.
>
> If I can find the courage to come to a place of honesty... my heart hurts. It hurts so much that I feel it could burst and I would never recover. I try so hard to be strong, push the emotions down, and move on. But that doesn't work for very long.
>
> I'm afraid to confront the pain I have bottled up for so long. I cavalierly say to others, "Yeah, we've lost two babies. We'll have children someday." The emotions are complicated. I don't resent others for having successful pregnancies at all. I celebrate with them for the huge accomplishment of having a baby. It's hard. The truth is that I am left with a gaping hole, and

I don't know what to do with it. God, I need Your help to start this healing process. Please hold my hand and guide me through it.

> *My grief is beyond healing; my heart is broken.*
>
> –Jeremiah 8:18

> *We are pressed on every side by troubles, but we are not crushed. We are perplexed, but not driven to despair. We are hunted down, but never abandoned by God. We get knocked down, but we are not destroyed. Through suffering, our bodies continue to share in the death of Jesus so that the life of Jesus may also be seen in our bodies.*
>
> *But we continue to preach because we have the same kind of faith the psalmist had when he said, "I believed in God, so I spoke." We know that God, who raised the Lord Jesus, will also raise us with Jesus and present us to himself together with you. All of this is for your benefit. And as God's grace reaches more and more people, there will be great thanksgiving, and God will receive more and more glory.*
>
> *That is why we never give up. Though our bodies are dying, our spirits are being renewed every day. For our present troubles are small and won't last very long. Yet they produce for us a glory that vastly outweighs them and will last forever! So we don't look at the troubles we can see now; rather, we fix our gaze on things that cannot be seen. For the things we see now will soon be gone, but the things we cannot see will last forever.*
>
> – 2 Corinthians 4:8–10, 13–18

Journal Entry from July 16, 2011:

The last full journal that I completed was filled with high hopes and grave disappointments, some heartaches that were just too painful to make reality on paper, and the occasional glimpse that God has not left me.

It has been quite the journey. As Lamentations 3:21 says, "Yet I still dare to hope." I'm not sure that I'm ready to hope again, but I am ready to trust God with the next step.

Hope is scary. I have seen it lead to disappointment too many times. But I know that God is good and faithful and unchanging. I know that God will never leave me no matter what life brings my way. Here's to trusting God with new adventures!

Journal Entry from October 12, 2011:

God, I know you're working on my heart. I am so afraid. Healing hurts so much. Please hold my hand and guide me through this process. I finally have the courage to ask You: What is the source of my depression and panic attacks? God, please reveal the source of my pain. Maybe it's multiple things. Please show me.

> *Give all your worries and cares to God, for he cares about you.*
>
> – 1 Peter 5:7

> *In His kindness, God called you to His eternal glory by means of Jesus Christ. After you have suffered a little while, He will restore, support, and strengthen you, and He will place you on a firm foundation.*
>
> – 1 Peter 5:10

> *Do not be afraid or discouraged, for the Lord is the one who goes before you. He will be with you; He will neither fail you nor forsake you.*
>
> – Deuteronomy 31:8

> *He gives power to those who are tired and worn out; He offers strength to the weak.*
>
> – Isaiah 40:29

> *Each time he said, 'My gracious favor is all you need. My power works best in your weakness.' So now I am glad to boast about my weakness, so that the power of Christ may work through me. Since I know it is all for Christ's good, I am quite content with my weakness and with insults, hardships, persecutions, and calamities. For when I am weak, then I am strong.*
>
> – 2 Corinthians 12:9–10

I have lost two babies. I'm not sure what to do with that. My heart has been ripped out of my chest twice. How do I hope again? How do I recover? How do I heal?

The song "All of Me" by Matt Hammitt has been such an encouragement to me. His testimony is so powerful. And the lyrics remind me that when fear, sadness, and brokenness are fighting for my attention, I can be brave and trust God with all of me.

I was wondering where to start. Then I realized that the way forward starts with surrender. I am terrified when I consider how much I have to lose. My heart hurts so much; I can't afford to lose any more. Another loss would break me. God, help me to surrender.

GO DEEPER

In this section, I reference Sarah's story of barrenness and lack of belief in God's promise. Go deeper and read Genesis 18:1–15, Genesis 21:1–6, and Hebrews 11:11 to discover the power of God's word and fulfilled promises despite impossible circumstances.

Coming to a place where I could acknowledge my need to surrender was crucial. It helped me to continue to choose hope. I clung to stories in the Bible in which women of faith like Sarah and Hannah had experienced similar circumstances. Having babies was completely out of their control.

Abraham and Sarah's story offered a lifeline of hope for me. God had given Abraham a promise that he would become the father of a multitude of nations. (Genesis 17:4) However, Abraham's wife was not able to get pregnant. The Bible describes Sarah's condition as barren. Merriam-Webster defines barren as, "not producing or incapable of producing offspring; sterile; unproductive; unfruitful; bleak; lifeless." For Abraham and Sarah, it wasn't about just a couple of years of trying. It had been decades of trying to get pregnant with no result. God's promise seemed impossible, especially when Sarah was 90 years old, and Abraham was 100 years old. In Sarah's mind, this was a done deal. There was no reason to hope any longer. Her body was well past the years of being able to have children. I love how God's word supersedes physical bounds.

Genesis 18:9 –15:

> *"Where is Sarah, your wife?" they asked him.*
>
> *"In the tent," Abraham replied.*
>
> *Then one of them said, "About this time next year I will return, and your wife, Sarah, will have a son!"*
>
> *Now Sarah was listening to this conversation from the tent nearby. And since Abraham and Sarah were both very old, and Sarah was long past the age of having children, she laughed silently to herself. "How could a*

worn-out woman like me have a baby?" she thought. "And when my master—my husband—is also so old?"

Then the LORD said to Abraham, "Why did Sarah laugh? Why did she say, 'Can an old woman like me have a baby?' Is anything too hard for the LORD? About a year from now I will return, and Sarah will have a son."

Sarah was afraid, so she denied that she had laughed. But he said, "That is not true. You did laugh."

I appreciate that Sarah laughed. I can only imagine what must have been going through her mind when she heard she would have a baby. I'm sure her heart was tempted to hope that it could be true, but you can hear that disbelief and doubt with her question of "How could a worn-out woman like me have a baby?" But it's humbling when God calls her out regarding her laughter at the idea of having a baby. She denies that she laughed out of fear. I'm really glad that God said something to her. It was His loving way of reminding her to expand her faith, think bigger, and give more room for God to work. My own heart fills with expectation and hope at God's response, "Is anything too hard for the LORD?" I have to remind myself to give God more room to work. I find that my expectations are often too small or limiting.

The LORD kept his word and did for Sarah exactly what he had promised. She became pregnant, and she gave birth to a son for Abraham in his old age. This happened at the time God had said it would.

– Genesis 21:1–2

It was by faith that even Sarah together was able to have a child, though she was barren and too old. She believed that God would keep his promise.

– Hebrews 11:11

God's word carries so much power. If He can make a way for 90-year-old Sarah to get pregnant and have a son, I can choose to trust God with my ability (or lack thereof) to have babies—even if it seems impossible. When God speaks, every detail of what He says happens. He was faithful to keep His promise to Sarah, and I can trust in that same faithfulness.

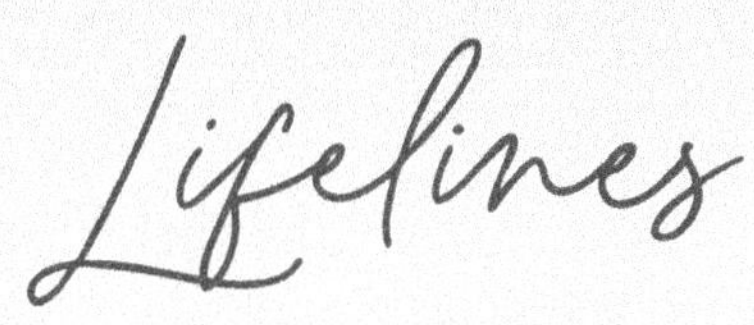

QUESTIONS TO CONSIDER

Even the Bible says in Proverbs 13:12a, "Hope deferred makes the heart sick." How does your heart respond to repeated events of loss or disappointment?

What do you do when your circumstances contradict God's promises?

SCRIPTURE VERSES

When you go through deep waters, I will be with you. When you go through rivers of difficulty, you will not drown. When you walk through the fire of oppression, you will not be burned up; the flames will not consume you. For I am the LORD, your god, the Holy One of Israel, your Savior. I gave Egypt as a ransom for your freedom; I gave Ethiopia and Seba in your place. – Isaiah 43:2–3

My grief is beyond healing; my heart is broken. – Jeremiah 8:18

Give all your worries and cares to God, for He cares about you. – 1 Peter 5:7

He gives power to the weak and strength to the powerless." – Isaiah 40:29

WORSHIP SONGS

"All of Me" by Matt Hammitt from his *Every Falling Tear* album.

"You Know Me" by Steffany Gretzinger from the *The Loft Sessions* album.

"What I Know" by Tricia from her *Radiate* album.

QUOTES

"What gives me the most hope every day is God's grace; knowing that his grace is going to give me the strength for whatever I face, knowing that nothing is a surprise to God." - Rick Warren[6]

"As I'm sure you already know, fear is an insidious force that has silenced the dreams and sabotaged the development of so many of God's children. But activating this confession gives us access to a much greater force—the counter-active force of faith: God says He will." - Steven Furtick (emphasis added)[7]

"Little fears can cohabitate and combine to form levels of anxiety and terror that will annihilate our awareness of the presence of God. I love the way the Amplified Bible translates 1 John 4:18: There is no fear in love [dread does not exist], but full-grown (complete, perfect) love turns fear out of doors and expels every trace of terror!" - Steven Furtick[8]

BOOKS

Crash the Chatterbox by Steven Furtick.

PRAYER

God, I pray against any lies the enemy may be trying to speak into my friends' hearts and minds right now. Cause them to dive deeper into Your word to hear Your voice and silence the voice of the enemy with Your truth. Remind my dear friends how strong they are in You. The enemy uses fear as a last resort when nothing else is working. Allow them to see that victory is in their grasp. Thank You, Jesus, for healing and making Your presence known in this season. Amen.

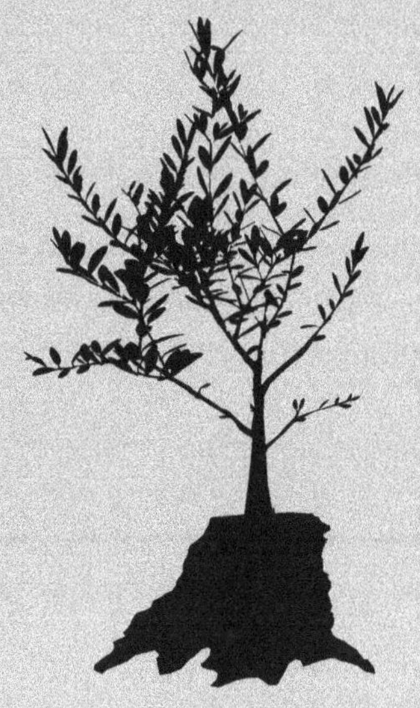

GOD SAID...

I have a promise for you.

The Promise

Let all that I am wait quietly before God,
for my hope is in him. – Psalm 62:5

GOD'S TIMING IS A ROUGH THING TO WRAP MY MIND AROUND. I frequently wish I could get a download of His five-year plan for my life or for even the next seven days. It would be nice to get a sneak peek at how long it might take for prayers to be answered. But God is wise in that way. If I were to see fully what the future held, I might feel overwhelmed at how big it is or be tempted to give up knowing that the future version of me feels impossible right now. In many cases, ignorance truly is bliss. But waiting is the worst!

In the middle of our waiting, Flip woke up one morning and told me about a dream or vision he had to open a coffee shop. He could see the logo of his business and how he could impact many people with the greater calling of sharing Jesus through coffee. Flip was in the process of pursuing his calling to open a coffee shop when, by a fun series of seemingly random events, we met a wonderful woman named Shawn at a local craft fair. She was selling one-pound bags of coffee for her nonprofit called Coffee4Kids Honduras to help support a children's hospital in San Pedro Sula, Honduras. All the coffee was locally grown in Honduras. We hit it off right away and soon found ourselves joining one of her regular mission trips to Honduras. We made arrangements to join Shawn in Honduras a week early in order to visit the local coffee farm and meet the family that has run it for generations. It was breathtaking and unforgettable. What a legacy they have built. They hand-sort all the good coffee beans from the bad ones. Their dedication to their craft is truly admirable. The other local coffee farms in the area work with this family to roast and sell their beans as well.

A couple of weeks before we left for Honduras, we discovered we were pregnant and cautiously celebrated a new life. We were only able to celebrate this sweet life for six weeks as I miscarried naturally three days before we were scheduled to board a plane to Honduras. I seriously considered whether I should I still go.

Journal Entries from September 2, 2013:

Why does fear come so easy? Something beautiful and amazing can happen, yet my mind defaults to thoughts of fear and "What-ifs."

I took a pregnancy test on Friday, August 30, 2013, and it was positive. It seemed like my period was a little late, which is abnormal. I was having drastic mood swings ranging from rage to sobbing for no reason. PMS for me is normally asking my husband if he is mad at me. I was also feeling really dizzy and slightly nauseous. My good friend, Crystal, took me to Wal-Mart and bought me prenatals and two pregnancy tests. Turns out, we're pregnant! We haven't said a word to anyone yet.

I've been calling midwives this week and setting up free consultations. It's so easy for me to be concerned and not trust my body to carry this little life to term. This has been a year of God's favor, and I'm pleading that this little four-week-old will be able to thrive in these next couple crucial months. We're unemployed and uninsured and pregnant—not only expecting a baby but also opening a coffee shop. It all seems crazy and impossible. But thankfully we serve a God who has slain the impossible. We serve the same God who raised Jesus from the dead. Nothing is impossible for God.

Journal Entries from September 11, 2013:

Nothing is impossible for you, God! You raised Jesus from the dead. You perform miracles. You heal the sick. You breathe life into our frail forms. Thank You for Your goodness and faithfulness. You are so holy and worthy of praise!

Holy Spirit, please touch my baby and cause our little baby to grow and thrive. Please cause all these cells to form correctly. Touch its little body while its hands and feet and eyes and heart are being formed.

I'm afraid, but I choose to trust You and believe that You will bless us with a child. I ask in faith that You give me a picture of hope.

> *And I am convinced that nothing can ever separate us from God's love. Neither death nor life, neither angels nor demons, neither our fears for*

> *today nor our worries about tomorrow—not even the powers of hell can separate us from God's love.*
>
> – Romans 8:38

I then wrote the shortest and most pointed journal entry to date. These three words carried with them a lot of weight.

> Journal Entries from September 13, 2013:
>
> I miscarried today.

You know it's a bad day when only three words make it into the journal. My heart was incredibly heavy, and I wasn't really sure how to pull it all together and serve others on a mission trip in another country. While my body was still healing, we headed to San Pedro Sula, Honduras. We connected with the lovely family running the coffee farm and then met up with the rest of the team to provide medical supplies to local families at a day camp. Then we spent a full week of loving on kids and running adult VBS (Vacation Bible School) at the local children's hospital. I asked the mission team what in the world adult VBS was. I learned that it's an hour dedicated to parents who have children suffering trials such as diseases, cancer, and burns. I was asked to lead one of the sessions that week. I sat down the night before and out poured six pages of testimony and hope. Having lost our third baby, my heart broke for these parents who were feeling hopeless for their precious babies too. It is truly remarkable to me what God is able to accomplish when you are willing to take a single step of courage and share your heart. Here is the testimony I shared with the parents that day.

> Testimony to Honduran Parents from November 4, 2013:
>
> I want to share a story with you about stones of remembrance. A stone of remembrance is an object that helps you to remember God's promises or a moment of God's goodness in your life. It is so important to remember these moments.
>
> The Bible mentions several times about stone pillars or altars being set up as a way to remember acts of God.
>
> *Jacob set up a stone pillar to mark the place where God had spoken to him. Then he poured wine over it as an offering to God and anointed the pillar with olive oil. And Jacob named the place Bethel (which means "house of God"), because God had spoken to him there.*
>
> – Genesis 35:14–15

So Joshua called together the twelve men he had chosen—one from each of the tribes of Israel. He told them, "Go into the middle of the Jordan, in front of the Ark of the LORD your God. Each of you must pick up one stone and carry it out on your shoulder—twelve stones in all, one for each of the twelve tribes of Israel. We will use these stones to build a memorial. In the future your children will ask you, 'What do these stones mean?' Then you can tell them, 'They remind us that the Jordan River stopped flowing when the Ark of the LORD's Covenant went across.' These stones will stand as a memorial among the people of Israel forever."

–Joshua 4:4–7

Joshua recorded these things in the Book of God's Instructions. As a reminder of their agreement, he took a huge stone and rolled it beneath the terebinth tree beside the Tabernacle of the LORD. Joshua said to all the people, "This stone has heard everything the LORD said to us. It will be a witness to testify against you if you go back on your word to God."

–Joshua 24:26–27

Many times, we pray and pray and ask for God's help or healing or blessing. But what happens when He answers our prayers? What happens when we receive healing or blessing? God deserves the glory and honor and praise. It's good to remember. It's easy to focus on the bad things that happen in our lives. With sickness or death or painful circumstances, it can be easy to lose sight of God and feel hopeless. That's why we need tangible reminders of God's goodness in our lives. We need something to hold onto.

I have a story for you that I have not shared with anyone before today. In 2006, my husband and I found out that we were pregnant and going to have a baby. We were overjoyed. So excited. We told our family and friends and started planning and picking names. At twelve weeks, we went to the doctor for a routine visit. The doctor looked at us and said there was no heartbeat, and that our baby was no longer alive. We were devastated and heartbroken. We sat in that room in silence and just wept. We had believed we were going to have a baby. The loss was difficult news to accept.

Our friends didn't know what to say or how to encourage us. They would say, "Miscarriages are common. You'll have another baby." Their words didn't comfort me. I was not ready to hope for another baby. I wanted the one I had lost.

One friend did help my heart to heal. She gave me a figurine of a child holding a wire balloon that said "HOPE" on the inside. She told me,

"Don't forget that you had a life inside you. This figurine will give you something to hold onto and allow you to remember." It was a tremendous encouragement to me.

Five years later, my husband and I found out we were pregnant again. We were very excited, but also nervous about possibly losing this one as well. When we went to the doctor at seven weeks into the pregnancy, the news was not good. Again, there was no heartbeat in our baby. I felt so empty and broken. When I lost this one, I was able to hold it briefly. It was the size of my pinky finger, and I could see a little head and hands and feet. For that brief moment, I got a glimpse of the miracle of life, and it was beautiful. God allowed me to hold onto hope for a little longer.

Last month, we found out we were pregnant again. We were quietly excited but afraid to hope. Daily I was praying and asking for God's blessing. I had a friend ask me, "No matter what happens, do you trust God?" And I said, "Yes. I trust God." Three days before coming to Honduras, we lost our third baby at six weeks into the pregnancy. While I am grieving on the inside, I have to stop, and say, "I know that my God is good. I know that my God is always with me. I know that He comforts me. My God is faithful. And He loves me."

I don't tell you these stories to make you sad. I want to share with you that in the midst of loss and pain and grieving, there is hope. My God loves me, and He loves our babies and children. I know that He is holding my precious babies in Heaven. I am so grateful for those precious weeks that I got to carry those little lives inside me.

I remembered that God lost His son too. He knows the pain I feel. His only son died. God knows the pain of loss. His love for us is so great that He was willing to send His only son, Jesus, to die and then be raised again, so that we could become part of His family.
If you don't know God and would like to become part of His family today, you can repeat this prayer after me.

> God, I want to become part of Your family. Please come into my life. Forgive me for the mistakes I've made. Please heal the pain in my heart. I choose to trust You with my life. Thank You for loving me. In Jesus' name, Amen.

NOTHING IS IMPOSSIBLE FOR GOD

> *Through their faith, the people in days of old earned a good reputation. By faith we understand that the entire universe was formed at God's*

> *command, that what we now see did not come from anything that can be seen... It was by faith that Noah built a large boat to save his family from the flood. He obeyed God, who warned him about things that had never happened before. By his faith Noah condemned the rest of the world, and he received the righteousness that comes by faith.*
>
> *It was by faith that Abraham obeyed when God called him to leave home and go to another land that God would give him as his inheritance. He went without knowing where he was going. And even when he reached the land God promised him, he lived there by faith—for he was like a foreigner, living in tents. And so did Isaac and Jacob, who inherited the same promise. Abraham was confidently looking forward to a city with eternal foundations, a city designed and built by God. It was by faith that even Sarah was able to have a child, though she was barren and was too old. She believed that God would keep his promis... It was by faith that Isaac promised blessings for the future to his sons, Jacob and Esau. It was by faith that Jacob, when he was old and dying, blessed each of Joseph's sons and bowed in worship as he leaned on his staff.*
>
> *It was by faith that Joseph, when he was about to die, said confidently that the people of Israel would leave Egypt. He even commanded them to take his bones with them when they left... How much more do I need to say? It would take too long to recount the stories of the faith of Gideon, Barak, Samson, Jephthah, David, Samuel, and all the prophets. By faith these people overthrew kingdoms, ruled with justice, and received what God had promised them. They shut the mouths of lions, quenched the flames of fire, and escaped death by the edge of the sword. Their weakness was turned to strength. They became strong in battle and put whole armies to flight.*
>
> – Hebrews 11:2–3, 7–11, 20–22, 32–34

I brought stones with me today, so that you could take a moment and write one word on a stone that would help you to remember God's work in your life. I wrote the word Hope on my stone. I remembered Isaiah 26:3–4, so I wrote that verse reference on the bottom of my stone.

> *You will keep in perfect peace all who trust in you, all whose thoughts are fixed on you! Trust in the LORD always, for the LORD GOD is the eternal Rock.*
>
> – Isaiah 26:3–4

God, I ask for Your blessings and favor on these men and women. Thank You for Your goodness. Thank You for loving us and promising to be with us always. Amen.

> *I pray that from his glorious, unlimited resources he will empower you with inner strength through his Spirit. Then Christ will make his home in your hearts as you trust in him. Your roots will grow down into God's love and keep you strong. And may you have the power to understand, as all God's people should, how wide, how long, how high, and how deep his love is. May you experience the love of Christ, though it is too great to understand fully. Then you will be made complete with all the fullness of life and power that comes from God. Now all glory to God, who is able, through his mighty power at work within us, to accomplish infinitely more than we might ask or think. Glory to him in the church and in Christ Jesus through all generations forever and ever! Amen.*
>
> – Ephesians 3:16–21
>
> *He will cover you with his feathers. He will shelter you with his wings. His faithful promises are your armor and protection.*
>
> – Psalm 91:4

It was difficult to be that transparent with that group of parents when my pain was still so raw and fresh. But I learned what God can do with obedience. Every one of those parents that day asked Jesus to come into their lives. We prayed and cried together. I had the beautiful privilege of getting to share the hope I carry through Jesus with those parents.

SEEN BY GOD

After my husband and I returned home from Honduras, I felt despair creep in. We had experienced our third miscarriage, and I desperately needed hope and something to cling to. I was reading through Exodus during my quiet time with God, and I reread the story of the ten plagues. Super uplifting passage, right? Nothing like locusts and water turning to blood to lift your spirits. But reading through the ten plagues caught my attention. I noticed a trend as I read through the details of each plague.

"Then the LORD said…," These words appear in Exodus 7:1, 7:8, 7:14, 7:19; 8:1, 8:5, 8:16, 8:20; 9:1, 9:8, 9:13; 10:1, 10:12, 10:21; 11:1

"And the LORD did just as he had said," or *"just as the LORD had predicted,"* appears in Exodus 7:13, 7:22; 8:12, 8:13, 8:14, 8:24, 8:35; 9:6, 9:12, 9:19

God outlined what would take place, and it happened exactly as He said to the very last detail every time. God even gave specific instructions to the Israelites on how to spare their firstborn children, while Pharaoh and Egypt suffered. God spoke, and it happened just as He said. God spoke, and it happened. God spoke, and His word came to pass. God impressed upon my heart that He could be trusted to keep His word. In that moment, I asked God to give me a promise—something just for me.

When the Israelites were delivered from Egypt, God led them by a pillar of cloud during the day and a pillar of fire during the night. (Exodus 13:22) I wanted to have a promise from God that felt as tangible as He was to the Israelites during their journey to the Promised Land. With full belief that God would provide me with a promise of my own, I decided to close my Bible and let it fall open wherever it may. I immediately questioned this method and thought I might be losing my mind. I couldn't possibly believe that letting my Bible fall open randomly would somehow show me a personal promise from God. Playing it "safe," I went to the back of my Bible to the concordance to see if maybe a key word might stand out as significant. No luck there. So, I took a breath, closed my Bible, and let it fall open where it may. It fell open in the book of Psalms. Of course, it did! It's the middle of the Bible. I was quick to dismiss that there could possibly be a promise from God in the middle of Psalms; however, the Holy Spirit nudged me to look at where the pages had opened. On the upper left-hand side, I took notice of Psalm 113:9, which reads:

> *He gives the barren woman a home, so that she becomes a happy mother. Praise the LORD!*

I wept.

In that moment, I felt so totally and completely known by Almighty God. I have never once prayed or asked God for a home or children. These are the two things that my heart had longed for more than anything on the planet. Growing up, we always lived in borrowed spaces. We rented and lived out of a mechanic's garage. We lived with my aunt. We moved into my stepdad's house. I lived in a dorm at college. We lived with my dad. Having a home of my own, a safe place to nurture babies and others, would make my heart sing and dance. But I never once asked or prayed for a home in case it was not meant to be. I didn't want to be disappointed if my prayer was not answered. In the same way, I never asked for babies of my own in case it was not meant to be. The disappointment would kill me, so I remained quiet on the topic. Thankfully, God spoke and broke the silence, giving me this beautiful promise! In one single verse, He promised the two things my heart longed for most—having a home and becoming a mother. God's word can be trusted. He speaks, and creation is formed. He speaks, and life is conceived out of barrenness. He speaks, and it happens.

God heard the laments of my heart and my plea for a promise I could hold onto. Not only did he answer my prayer, but He also gave me three promises:

- He will give me, a barren woman, a home.
- I will become a happy or joyous mother.
- And these two promises carried with them an additional promise of hope for a future I had previously been afraid to utter out loud.

Lifelines

QUESTIONS TO CONSIDER

Have you taken the time to ask God for a specific promise just for you? Ask Him for a verse—a promise that you can hold onto and claim. Write it down on the lines below.

SCRIPTURE VERSES

Let us hold tightly without wavering to the hope we affirm, for God can be trusted to keep His promise. – Psalm 62:5

Testimonies of great faith in Hebrews. 11:2–3, 7–11, 20–22, 32–34

You will keep in perfect peace all who trust in you, all whose thoughts are fixed on you! Trust in the LORD always, for the LORD GOD is the eternal Rock. – Isaiah 26:3–4

I pray that from his glorious, unlimited resources he will empower you with inner strength through his Spirit. Then Christ will make his home in your hearts as you trust in him. Your roots will grow down into God's love and keep you strong. And may you have the power to understand, as all God's people should, how wide, how long, how high, and how deep his love is. May you experience the love of Christ, though it is too great to understand fully. Then you will be made complete with all the fullness of life and power that comes from God. Now all glory to God, who is able, through his mighty power at work within us, to accomplish infinitely more than we might ask or think. Glory to him in the church and in Christ Jesus through all generations forever and ever! Amen. – Ephesians 3: 16–21

He will cover you with his feathers. He will shelter you with his wings. His faithful promises are your armor and protection. – Psalm 91:4

WORSHIP SONGS

"It Is Well" by Kristene Dimarco from the *You Make Me Brave (Live)* album.

"Say the Word" by Hillsong UNITED from their *Empires* album.

"Thy Will" by Hillary Scott & The Scott Family from their *Love Remains* album.

"Known" by Tauren Wells from his *Hills and Valleys (Deluxe Edition)* album.

"Split the Sea" by Hannah Kerr.

"Promises" by Joe L Barnes, Naomi Raine from the *Maverick City Vol. 3 Part 1* album.

QUOTES

"True faith means holding nothing back. It means putting every hope in God's fidelity to His Promises." - Francis Chan[9]

"God never made a promise that was too good to be true." - Dwight L. Moody[10]

"The best praying man is the man who is most believingly familiar with the promises of God. After all, prayer is nothing but taking God's promises to him, and saying to him, "Do as thou hast said." Prayer is the promise utilized. A prayer which is not based on a promise has no true foundation." - Charles Spurgeon[11]

"God is able to take the mess of our past and turn it into a message. He takes the trials and tests and turns them into a testimony." - Christine Caine[12]

BOOKS

Undaunted: Daring to Do What God Calls You to Do by Christine Caine

PRAYER

God, Your word is powerful! Everything You say will come to pass. You are faithful to keep Your promises. Fear, doubt, hopelessness, anxiety, and lies from the enemy can all take a hike. God, You are so good. We praise You in advance for answered prayers and fulfilled promises. In Jesus' undisputed name, Amen.

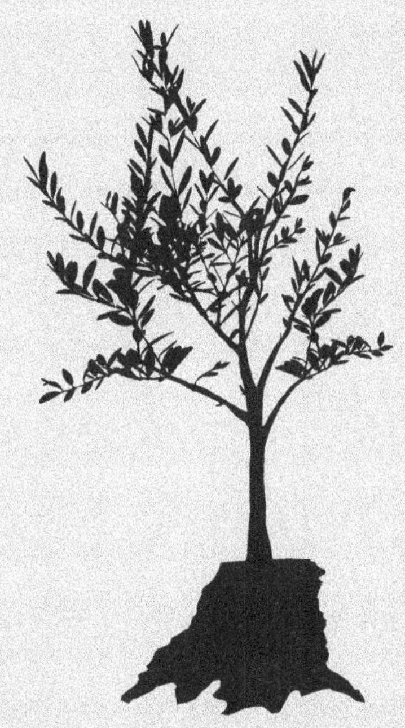

GOD SAID... *trust.*

Choosing Trust

If God can bring blessing from the broken body of Jesus and glory from something that's as obscene as the cross, He can bring blessing from my problems and my pain and my unanswered prayer. I just have to trust Him. – Anne Graham Lotz

TIME CAN BE CRUEL. I hear in my head the familiar saying, "Time heals all wounds." After three miscarriages, my heart strongly disagreed, and my thoughts immediately reflected a scenario where I shoot the messenger. My heart had not healed. Instead, I carried compounded grief and anguish inside. The weight of it was suffocating.

God's promise to me in Psalm 113:9 poked a hole through my darkness and gave me renewed fuel to hope again. Taking things one day at a time, I dove into Scripture. I couldn't get enough. Stories that I'd read previously were coming to life. It should have been obvious, but I was discovering that these Bible stories were personal testimonies about the faithfulness of God given by real people. As I read more and more, it was reassuring to know that others have experienced similar pain and that I could trust God with it all.

One such story in 1 Samuel caught my attention. Hannah and I would have been great friends. First Samuel 1:2–2:21 tells us that Hannah was married to a man named, Elkanah. "Elkanah had two wives, Hannah and Peninnah. Peninnah had children, but Hannah did not." (1 Samuel 1:2) You can already see where this is going. Every year it was customary for them to travel to Shiloh to worship and offer sacrifices to the Lord. Elkanah would give portions of the meat to Peninnah and her children, and then only one portion to Hannah. Hannah felt her longing for children even more deeply when she received her single portion. To make matters worse, Peninnah would taunt Hannah often reducing her to tears.

One year, Hannah finally had it. She couldn't take it anymore; she felt that her heart might burst if she could not have children of her own. She went into the Temple.

> *Hannah was in deep anguish, crying bitterly as she prayed to the LORD. And she made this vow: "O LORD of Heaven's Armies, if you will look upon my sorrow and answer my prayer and give me a son, then I will give him back to you. He will be yours for his entire lifetime, and as a sign that he has been dedicated to the Lord, his hair will never be cut."*
> – 1 Samuel 1:10–11

As she was praying to God out of great anguish and sorrow, the priest saw her and thought she might be drunk. She assured him that she was pouring her heart out to God. The priest replied to her, "Go in peace! May the God of Israel grant the request you have asked of him." (1 Samuel 1:17)

A year later, Hannah's desperate prayer to God was answered just as the priest had told her. She gave birth to a son, dedicated him to God, and then God went above and beyond and blessed her with seven more children.

I love Hannah's heart and unapologetic desperation before God. She was so incredibly brave. With the miraculous answer to prayer, Hannah dedicated her firstborn son to God just as she had promised and gave her boy to the Temple to be raised by priests. I can't even imagine the courage that it took to leave her boy in the care of others. It wasn't until recently that I really learned more about who Samuel was to become. Samuel became the prophet who anointed King David. Yes, this is the same David who started as a shepherd and who fought and slayed the giant Goliath with a sling and rock. King David's lineage ultimately birthed Jesus, the Messiah, Son of God, Savior to the world. What a powerful

GO DEEPER

In this section, I reference Hannah's story of courageous prayer and faith for a child. Go deeper and read 1 Samuel 1:1–3:21, 7:15–8:22, 9:15–10:27, 13:1–16:13 to discover the power of faith and prayer. Read about how Samuel learns to hear the voice of God, courageously walks in his calling, and becomes the prophet who anoints King David. Wow! What a legacy from the heart cries of a believing woman.

legacy stemming from the prayers of a God-fearing woman who knew in her heart that she was meant to have children.

DESPERATE

Almost two years after our third loss and trip to Honduras, we welcomed a fourth pregnancy with much trepidation. It is a complicated pile of emotions to hold onto the hope of God's promise, fear more loss, wrestle with existing grief, and force the courage to speak hope and life over a new pregnancy. When we received the positive pregnancy test, South Coast Midwifery (SCW) must have thought I was losing my mind when I called and pleaded to be put on progesterone immediately. I was desperate to hold onto this pregnancy and wanted to take every precaution. Hopefully, they blamed my overreaction and persistence on the pregnancy hormones coursing through my body.

> ### Journal Entries from May 4, 2015:
>
> On Sunday morning (May 3, 2015), we decided to take a pregnancy test. And it was as clear as day two dark blue lines—pregnant! We are both so excited, and it was fun to be able to share the news with Flip's parents who happened to be in town. I'm calling South Coast Midwifery today to set up a time to get progesterone this week.
>
> God, I am in awe at Your blessings and provisions. Thank You for Your hand of favor on our lives. Thank You for this precious little life growing inside me right now. I feel so blessed. Thank You for this joy I have welling up inside of me. Praise You, Jesus! Thank You, Holy Spirit, for planting in me unwavering hope that would not die.
>
> *I pray that God, the source of hope, will fill you completely with joy and peace because you trust in him. Then you will overflow with confident hope through the power of the Holy Spirit.*
>
> – Romans 15:13

> ### Journal Entries from May 5, 2015:
>
> *Fear of the LORD is the foundation of wisdom. Knowledge of the Holy One results in good judgment.*
>
> – Proverbs 9:10
>
> I will not let fear win or control me. This baby inside me is an amazing gift from God whether I get to hold him or not. God, I choose to trust You. I will not let circumstances manipulate or control my emotions.

> He whispers in my ear and tells me that I'm fearless. I am all that He says I am. Holy Spirit, please break off this fear and panic from me in Jesus' powerful name. I am free.

> Journal Entries from May 8, 2015:
>
> *You haven't done this before. Ask, using my name, and you will receive, and you will have abundant joy.*
>
> –John 16:24
>
> Thank you for the baby growing inside me. Five weeks strong. I heard from SCW that my progesterone levels were at 15.2 and should be about 20. They said not to worry and that they have seen lower levels. So, it was perfect timing getting on progesterone when I did. Thank You, Jesus, for protecting our baby in the meantime. The heart starts beating this week.

This little fighter made it to nine weeks in the womb. This is not where I tell you how God's presence washed all the pain away, and I magically mustered the courage to push through this loss and get pregnant right away. Nope. I was completely wrecked. God had just given me His word and promise in Psalm 113:9 that I would have a home and become a joyous mother. This was the time to see His promise fulfilled and hold a sweet baby of our own in our arms. But instead, I felt myself sink into depression and withdraw a bit. God made us, as humans, to be mind, body, will, and emotions. In order to survive and not completely lose it, my body shut my emotions down. I didn't have a way to process or understand this level of grief. It was all out of my control. I could have easily been angry at God and shut Him out completely. But I wasn't mad at God. I wasn't angry at all. I was numb. I blamed myself. I felt completely defeated. I felt broken.

Baby number four. Sigh. At the time, my every exhale resulted in tears. My state of mind kinda looked like this...

> If my daily interactions don't go e-x-a-c-t-l-y according to plan right now, a full-blown panic attack and a deluge of tears will result. Everything feels so out of control that I don't have the capacity or patience to deal with anything else. This means I can't burn the toast for breakfast, run out of coffee, or shrink my shirt in the laundry right now. And above all else, please do not ask me how I'm doing.

With a complete meltdown on the verge, my thoughtful mother-in-law paid for us to get away and stay at the Marriott resort in Dana Point, California. The morning we woke up at the Marriott resort, I wandered down to the resort lounge, ordered a cup of Italian roast coffee, and sat by a big window with ocean and marina views. I could feel the warmth of the sunshine like a hug. The light poured in through the windows and highlighted my Bible and journal sitting there. I opened my journal to write as I have always done, but I didn't want to write. I couldn't write. I longed for this to be a bad stress dream and to wake up and find God's promise fulfilled. Ugh! I couldn't write, so I started listening to music. Lauren Daigle's song "First" had just come out. Every lyric felt like it was speaking straight to my fragile heart.

Journal Entries from June 4, 2015:

I barely have the courage to write. This is the part I dread the most—the finality of when truth hits paper. It's right there in front of me, plain as day. It's not just in my head anymore. It's not a fear or a bad dream—it's reality. We've lost our fourth baby at nine weeks.

As I sit here unable to speak or write, the song "First" by Lauren Daigle plays through my headphones giving me the words for this exact moment: "Before I speak a word, let me hear Your voice."[13]

I could journal about my fears of the future, but God Your love is loyal. You can be trusted to keep Your promises. I choose You and the plan You have for our lives. I will not be defeated. I ask that You please hold my tender heart in Your hands. Protect it from being darkened by grief, anger, and depression. Instead, please surround it with deep joy, love, and hope. I am an overcomer in Jesus Christ. I will be known by my persistent joy, not by bitterness or anger. I choose joy, because I have a promise from Almighty God!

> *Give thanks to the LORD, for he is good! His faithful love endures forever.*
>
> – Psalm 107:1

> *My heart is confident in you, O God; no wonder I can sing your praises Wake up, my soul!*
>
> – Psalm 108:1

> *The Lord's loved ones are precious to him; it grieves Him when they die.*
>
> – Psalm 116:15 NLT

God, You are the rock on which I stand. You are the God who parted waters. I will trust in You.

> *How joyful are those who fear the LORD—all who follow his ways! You will enjoy the fruit of your labor. How joyful and prosperous you*

> *will be! Your wife will be like a fruitful grapevine, flourishing within your home. Your children will be like vigorous young olive trees as they sit around your table. That is the LORD's blessing for those who fear him.*
>
> – Psalm 128:1–4

Four pregnancies. Four times hoping for my body to work like it's supposed to—to bring life into this world. As a confession, I had to shut down my heart for a season. It was too painful to feel. Numbness was preferred.

> We cannot selectively numb emotions. When we numb the painful emotions, we also numb the positive emotions.
> - Brené Brown[14]

Unfortunately, one of the repercussions of choosing numbness meant choosing to avoid connection with others as well. It was a risk I had to take because my heart was too fragile to embrace vulnerability... yet.

I had to declare the following truths over and over again in this season. I read Scripture out loud. I kept reading Psalm 113:9, God's promise to me, over and over again until my heart had the courage to continue to believe in it:

- God is good.
- I, thankfully, have the ability to get pregnant.
- I am a mother even if I have not been able to hold my babies in my arms.
- Hope is not gone.

Lifelines

QUESTIONS TO CONSIDER

When the outcome looks bleak and everything is coming against you, can you trust that God is still in control? Why or why not?

Vent to God and ask Him for hope in your specific season or situation.

SCRIPTURE VERSES

The LORD's loved ones are precious to him; it grieves Him when they die. – Psalm 116:15

I pray that God, the source of hope, will fill you completely with joy and peace because you trust in him. Then you will overflow with confident hope through the power of the Holy Spirit. – Romans 15:13

The LORD is close to the brokenhearted; He rescues those whose spirits are crushed. The righteous person faces many troubles, but the LORD comes to the rescue each time." – Psalm 34:18–19)

I pray that from his glorious, unlimited resources he will empower you with inner strength through his Spirit. Then Christ will make his home in your hearts as you trust in him. Your roots will grow down into God's love and keep you strong. And may you have the power to understand, as all God's people should, how wide, how long, how high, and how deep his love is. May you experience

the love of Christ, though it is too great to understand fully. Then you will be made complete with all the fullness of life and power that comes from God. Now all glory to God, who is able, through his mighty power at work within us, to accomplish infinitely more than we might ask or think. Glory to him in the church and in Christ Jesus through all generations forever and ever! Amen.
– Ephesians 3: 16–21

He will cover you with his feathers. He will shelter you with his wings. His faithful promises are your armor and protection. – Psalm 91:4

WORSHIP SONGS

"First" by Lauren Daigle from her *How Can It Be* album.

"Letting Go" by Steffany Gretzinger from her *The Undoing* album.

"You Know Me" by Steffany Gretzinger from *The Loft Sessions* album.

"You Are My Champion" by Dante Bowe from the *Champion (Live)* album.

QUOTES

"We cannot selectively numb emotions. When we numb the painful emotions, we also numb the positive emotions." - Brené Brown[15]

"If God can bring blessing from the broken body of Jesus and glory from something that's as obscene as the cross, He can bring blessing from my problems and my pain and my unanswered prayer. I just have to trust Him." - Anne Graham Lotz[16]

PRAYER

God, nothing is a surprise to You. When we don't have answers and can't seem to see the light, You are still there. We trust You with the future and come to You with desperate prayers as Hannah did. Please hold us and continue to speak truth into our hearts and minds through Your word and the encouragement of other believers. Thank You for hearing our prayers and coming to our rescue. You are faithful and good. We choose to trust despite what our emotions may be screaming. In Jesus' name, Amen.

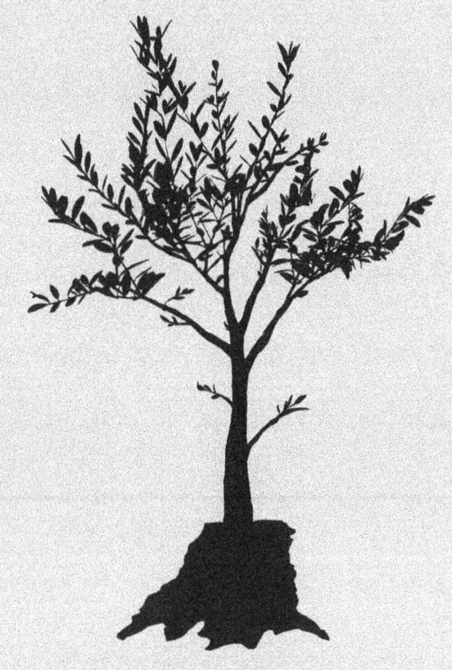

GOD SAID...

My mercies are new every morning.

Daring to Hope

I will never forget this awful time, as I grieve over my loss. Yet I still dare to hope when I remember this: The love of the Lord never ends! By his mercies we have been kept from complete destruction. Great is his faithfulness; his mercies begin afresh each day. – Lamentations 3:20–23

I WAS SITTING AT MY DESK WORKING ONE AFTERNOON. It was about two thirty, and I had a meeting coming up in the next thirty minutes. I was responding to some emails. I remember God interrupting me with this vision and asking me to draw a picture. The request was clear as day. On the left side of this picture, there was a dead, dried out tree in the middle of a barren wilderness. The tree had bare, gnarly branches; there were no leaves or signs of life. The ground was cracked and dry—only dust and wilderness all around. And then in the middle of this picture was a deep, deep pit. It was as if the pit had no end—just deep, endless darkness. I was sitting on the edge of the pit with my feet dangling looking down as far as I could see. I couldn't see anything but darkness. I felt the weight of my sadness and everything we had been through with our losses.

To the right side of the picture was another tree. It was full of life with fresh green leaves. There were even birds living among its branches. The ground around the tree was thick with lush green grass, and flowers were beginning to bloom. God reminded me that it's OK to remember where I've come from, but not to remain focused on it. He brought my attention to where I was sitting on the edge of the pit. I had drawn myself sitting on the right side of the pit with my feet dangling in and my head in my hands. I was looking down into the darkness and if I lifted my head, I could only see the bare, lifeless tree in the wilderness. God reminded me that I had already come through the wilderness and out of the pit. All I needed to do was turn around, get up, and walk in His blessings.

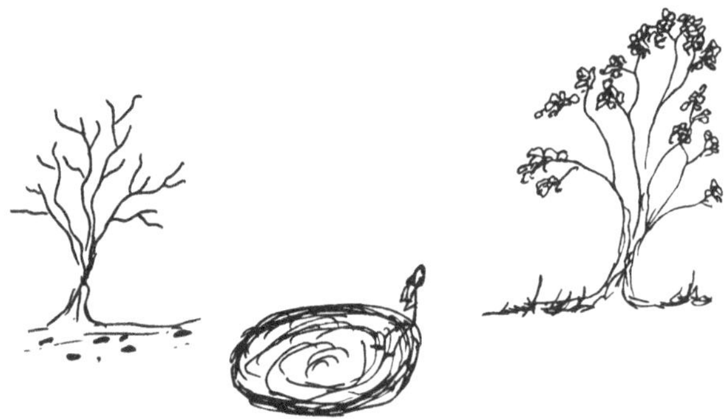

By 2015, my husband and I had experienced a lot of life. I was beginning to empathize more deeply with the apostle Paul than ever before. In 2 Corinthians 11, he describes a slew of hardships he had endured:

> *I have... been put in prison more often, been whipped times without number, and faced death again and again. Five different times the Jewish leaders gave me thirty-nine lashes. Three times I was beaten with rods. Once I was stoned. Three times I was shipwrecked. Once I spent a whole night and a day adrift at sea. I have traveled on many long journeys. I have faced danger from rivers and from robbers. I have faced danger from my own people, the Jews, as well as from the Gentiles. I have faced danger in the cities, in the deserts, and on the seas. And I have faced danger from men who claim to be believers but are not. I have worked hard and long, enduring many sleepless nights. I have been hungry and thirsty and have often gone without food. I have shivered in the cold, without enough clothing to keep me warm.*
>
> – 2 Corinthians 11:23–27

In eleven years of marriage, we had experienced:

- Four miscarriages.
- A fire in our storage unit that destroyed all our belongings, including Christmas decorations, my wedding dress, every letter Flip and I had written to each other while we were dating, all my oil paintings since eighth grade, and more.
- Four deaths among our extended family.
- Six years of intermittent employment and financial hardship.
- Anxiety and depression.

But through all this, like Paul, we learned what weakness really means and how to depend on God like never before.

> *Each time he said, "My grace is all you need. My power works best in*

> *weakness." So now I am glad to boast about my weakness, so that the power of Christ can work through me.*
>
> – 2 Corinthians 12:9

I'm grateful for reminders like this, because in this next season of life, I needed His strength more than ever.

> Journal Entries from August 25, 2015:
>
> It's amazing how much can happen in the course of a day. On the morning of my birthday, I took a pregnancy test. It was positive. Really fun birthday present.
>
> > *Those who listen to instruction will prosper; those who trust the LORD will be joyful.*
> >
> > – Proverbs 16:20
>
> > *But I trust in your unfailing love. I will rejoice because you have rescued me.*
> >
> > – Psalm 13:5

> Journal Entries from September 4, 2015:
>
> There have been a lot of ups and downs this week. I have had three sets of blood work done. The first one was positive with good HCG and progesterone levels. The second one showed a decline in HCG levels going from 890 down to 850. I took a third test yesterday, so I met with the doctor at eleven o'clock today to find out more.
>
> I keep talking to the baby and assuring him that he is loved and safe. And that no matter what he's in God's hands, even if I don't get to hold this baby personally. I trust God with my body, with my life, and with our baby's life.
>
> God, You are good.

> Journal Entries from September 4, 2015:
>
> We lost baby #5 yesterday. God, I am fighting thoughts that say, "I'm broken," or "Something is wrong with me."
>
> Dr. Cortez is starting a full workup for me to help identify what might be causing the premature losses. In six weeks, I will start testing that may or

may not be covered by insurance (mid-October).

God, please hold me close. The pain in my heart is big; it feels tangible. Please protect my heart in this time of grieving. Help me not to retreat inward. Help me to embrace my emotions and have the courage to face how I feel honestly. Protect me from shame and guilt.

God, please hold my babies and tell them that I love them each so dearly.

> *You will show me the way of life, granting me the joy of your presence and the pleasures of living with you forever.*
>
> – Psalm 16:11

I really like this passage from my devotional called "Healing Negative Emotions:

> Even though your circumstances may make you feel like you are walking through the valley of death, you will not fear because you know the Lord is with you. God's goodness toward you will be so visible that even your enemies will see His handiwork upon your life. They will see God's grace abounding toward you.[17]

> *But each day the LORD pours his unfailing love upon me, and through each night I sing his songs, praying to God who gives me life.*
>
> – Psalm 42:8

The song "You Set Me Free" by Angie Miller has been a huge encouragement recently reminding me that when I'm going through a storm and feeling weighed down, God's got me.

Journal Entries from September 21, 2015:

Help me, God. Please come to my rescue. My heart hurts more than I can bear. I grieve over my babies. I feel robbed. I feel such deep loss right now.

> *Your own ears will hear him. Right behind you a voice will say, "This is the way you should go," whether to the right or to the left.*
>
> – Isaiah 30:21

> *The LORD is close to the brokenhearted; he rescues those whose spirits are crushed. The righteous person faces many troubles, but the LORD comes to the rescue each time.*
>
> – Psalm 34:18–19 (emphasis added)

> *Take delight in the LORD, and he will give you your heart's desires. Commit everything you do to the LORD. Trust him, and he will help you.*
>
> – Psalm 37:4–5
>
> *Having hope will give you courage. You will be protected and will rest in safety.*
>
> –Job 11:18

> Journal Entries from October 8, 2015:
>
> I am now definitely showing signs of depression. It is a struggle to get up in the morning. I snooze four times. I just want to stay in bed and sleep and hide. I feel out of control. Our place is a disaster. Countertops are dirty. The floors are dirty. Every surface has something on it. I don't have any clean clothes right now because the laundry facility ruined six pieces of clothing last time. We can't afford to use it. So, I am reusing dirty underwear. I feel out of control.
>
> *Trust in the LORD always, for the LORD GOD is the eternal Rock.*
>
> – Isaiah 26:4
>
> I had a nightmare last night that all my dignity had been stripped. I was living in a place with no boundaries. Privacy was not respected. Showering without eyes watching was not an option. I had to remove myself (who I was) from my nakedness. There was no hiding.

As you can see from these journal entries, only a few months had passed before we were pregnant with baby number five. Our joy was short-lived as this little one was with us for only six weeks of pregnancy. To say that I was feeling defeated would be a gross understatement.

My doctor asked me if I had had any kind of workup done before. I let her know that my previous doctor advised us that we had to have at least three premature losses before they would order any tests to be done. With five premature losses at this point, we started the process of undergoing a full workup. Twelve blood tests were ordered, including hormone and genetics testing. We were cautioned that this level of in-depth testing could get pricey and that it's typically not covered by insurance. I was sincerely hoping to hear back with news about a hormone deficiency because I could take supplements and somehow ensure no future losses. It would be the easiest remedy.

> Journal Entries from March 17, 2016:
>
> I'm terrified to journal—partly because I don't know what the whole truth is yet. I heard back from Dr. Cortez about the blood results for the premature pregnancy losses. All my hormone levels are good. But the blood tests identified two genetic imbalances. She said I have two chromosomes that are borrowing an arm from each other. She said that this is what is causing the losses. She is referring us to the Fetal Diagnostics Center for a consultation to get more details on what this means and what our options are. She highly recommended that we not get pregnant right now to prevent additional losses. She is recommending IVF and wants me to be prepared to feel like a lab rat with all the tests, hormone injections, other procedures. I don't know what to feel. My spirit says, "Now God can work!" While my flesh and mind tell me I'm broken and can't have children.
>
> I told Flip as soon as he picked me up after work. We had a really nice dinner and decided we don't have enough info right now to make any big decisions. The consultation is scheduled for next Thursday, March 24 at eleven thirty.
>
> *For we live by believing and not by seeing.*
>
> – 2 Corinthians 5:7
>
> *For we live by faith, not by sight.*
>
> – 2 Corinthians 5:7 NIV

I should have been relieved and hopeful that my hormone levels came back normal. But getting confirmation that I have chromosomal translocation, a genetic disorder, was the last thing I wanted to hear from all the blood work that was done. You can take supplements to adjust and support hormone levels. You can't change your DNA. Our history of premature losses and this news of a genetic disorder suddenly took all hope out of my hands. It was official. When we asked Dr. Cortez if there were any additional tests we should take or if Flip should get tested, she said that there was no need to do any further testing because the test results confirmed the reason for the losses. There was literally nothing left to do now but continue to surrender and trust God to keep His promise.

> Journal Entries from March 28, 2016:
>
> After hearing about our test results, we met with a genetic counselor this past Thursday. We learned that I have Chromosomal Translocation. My #15 and #3 chromosomes share pieces with one another. I previously and ignorantly believed that any abnormalities with chromosomes automatical-

ly resulted in deformities or loss of function whether physically or mentally. While I am an intelligent, fully functioning person with all forty-six required chromosomes, my #15 and #3 chromosome situation make it challenging to reproduce. Each time I get pregnant, I have a fifty percent chance of having a healthy, fully developed baby, but we have been getting the other fifty percent each time so far. They left all decisions in our court. We can...

- Keep trying naturally and risk more losses.
- Pursue IVF where all the fertilization would happen in the lab. This would bypass the risk of additional miscarriages due to the chromosomal imbalance issue. They would select the healthy embryos and implant those and freeze the other healthy ones for later.
- Consider the third option, which is adoption.

It has been a lot to consider. I know that God is working through this. It isn't news to Him that I have Chromosomal Translocation. It's in my weakness that He gets all the glory. Now that I have this knowledge, God and I are on the same page.

My brain was swirling with both the finality of my condition and trusting God. With thoughts of despair and the unknown, I made a choice to choose hope, even though breakthrough was not yet evident. There was not yet any light at the end of the tunnel. I chose to reject the temptation to despair, and I held God to His word!

> *I will never forget this awful time, as I grieve over my loss. Yet I still dare to hope when I remember this: The unfailing love of the LORD never ends! His mercies never cease. Great is his faithfulness; his mercies begin afresh each morning.*
>
> – Lamentations 3:20–23

If God can grant Sarah and Abraham a son when they are nearly 100 years old, I can trust God to keep his promise to me: "I will give the barren woman a home, so that she will become a happy mother. Praise the Lord!" (Psalm 113:9)

> *The LORD kept his word and did for Sarah exactly what he had promised.*
>
> – Genesis 21:1

It was crucial during this time for me to read the truth of Scripture, write it down, and speak it out loud often. I needed the truth of His Word to be louder in my thoughts than the lies and temptation to despair of fighting for my hope. I quoted and prayed Psalm 113:9 back to God and pleaded with Him to be true to His word and keep His promise.

Lifelines

QUESTIONS TO CONSIDER

How do you respond when confronted with circumstances that are outside your control?

____

____

____

____

____

In what ways are you able to see God in the middle of your circumstances right now?

____

____

____

____

____

SCRIPTURE VERSES

I will never forget this awful time, as I grieve over my loss. Yet I still dare to hope when I remember this: The unfailing love of the LORD never ends! His mercies never cease. Great is his faithfulness; his mercies begin afresh each morning." – Lamentations 3:20–23

For we live by believing and not by seeing. – 2 Corinthians 5:7

Take delight in the LORD, and he will give you your heart's desires. Commit everything you do to the LORD. Trust him, and he will help you. – Psalm 37:4–5

Having hope will give you courage. You will be protected and will rest in safety. – Job 11:18

WORSHIP SONGS

"Cover the Earth (Live)" by Naomi Raine from *Cover The Earth (Live In New York)* album.

"You Set Me Free" by Angie Miller.

"Pieces" by Steffany Gretzinger from the *Have It All (Live)* album.

"Do it Again" by Elevation Worship from their *There is a Cloud* album.

"Have My Heart" by Chris Brown of Elevation Worship, Chandler Moore from the *Maverick City Vol. 3 Part 1* album.

SERMONS

"Hope In the Dark: Waiting on God" by Pastor Craig Groeschel, https://www.life.church/media/hope-in-the-dark/waiting-on-god

"Where Are You, God?" by Pastor Craig Groeschel, https://www.life.church/media/hope-in-the-dark/where-are-you-god

QUOTES

"Carve a tunnel of hope through the dark mountain of disappointment." - Martin Luther King Jr.[18]

"When we're suffering through hard times, we take God at his Word and believe that he's still in control, with a specific purpose in mind. So we keep going, relying on him. As we keep going, hour to hour, day to day, week to week, we become stronger. Our faith grows, our maturity grows, our trust in God grows. As we get stronger, we believe in God's goodness, more than our circumstances. We learn to believe in God's promises." - Craig Groeschel[19]

"Even as we cling to the promises of divine truth, we scrutinize our natural world for answers that require supernatural solutions. Somehow we inherently believe that if we can understand the motivation and contextualization of our crisis, then we can contain it, reduce it, and eliminate it." - Bishop T. D. Jakes[20]

BOOKS

Hope in the Dark by Craig Groeschel

PRAYER

God, please take all these broken pieces and unanswered questions that are haunting my mind. I can't possibly contend with the depth of my disappointment right now. You say that I am fearfully and wonderfully made (Psalm 139:13), and that I have a hope and a future. (Jeremiah 29:11) I am holding You to Your Word. Be with me and remind me that Your promises still hold true. You are God. Please take my hand and show me the next step. I need You. In Jesus' name, Amen.

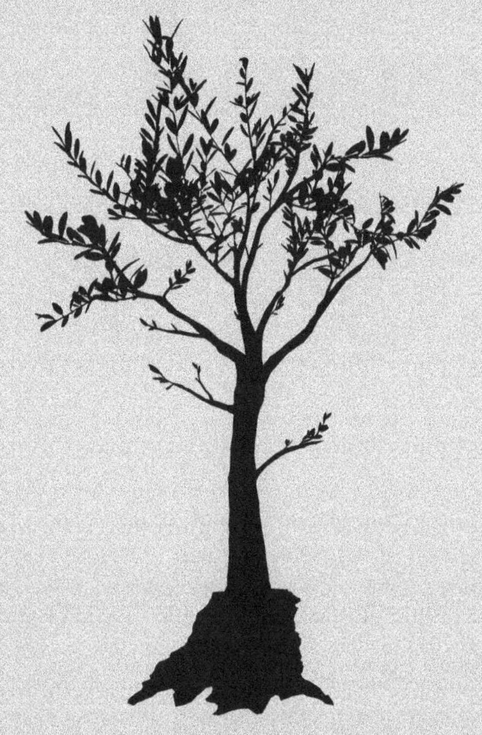

GOD SAID... *look up, I've got you.*

Nowhere but Up

I waited patiently for the LORD; he turned to me and heard my cry. He lifted me out of the slimy pit, out of the mud and mire; he set my feet on a rock and gave me a firm place to stand. He put a new song in my mouth, a hymn of praise to our God. Many will see and fear the LORD and put their trust in him. . - Psalm 40:1–3 NIV

WHEN THERE IS A PATTERN OR TREND OF LOSS, it becomes increasingly difficult to hope for a better outcome. I know that God gave me a promise in Psalm 113:9 that I would be given a home and become a joyous mother. I was holding Him to His word nearly every day—reciting it to myself, writing that promise down, and prayerfully repeating it back to God—as if He needed a reminder. But I received that promise right after our third loss. We had since endured three additional losses and received genetic results that I have chromosomal translocation. I felt lost and genuinely didn't know how to get out of the darkness I was living with. The only thing I knew was that God was the only one who could help.

CRYING OUT FOR RESCUE

I read through a lot of the book of Psalms and grew a new deep fondness for the relationship that King David had with God. For me, the book of Psalms was like getting ahold of David's private journals and reading his candid conversations with God. For example, Psalm 77:1–12 says:

> *I cry out to God; yes, I shout. Oh, that God would listen to me!*
>
> *When I was in deep trouble, I searched for the Lord.*
> *All night long I prayed, with hands lifted toward heaven, but my soul was not comforted.*

I think of God, and I moan, overwhelmed with longing for his help. You don't let me sleep. I am too distressed even to pray!

I think of the good old days, long since ended, when my nights were filled with joyful songs. I search my soul and ponder the difference now.

Has the Lord rejected me forever? Will he never again be kind to me? Is his unfailing love gone forever? Have his promises permanently failed? Has God forgotten to be gracious? Has he slammed the door on his compassion? And I said, "This is my fate; the Most High has turned his hand against me."

But then I recall all you have done, O LORD; I remember your wonderful deeds of long ago. They are constantly in my thoughts. I cannot stop thinking about your mighty works.

David is exhausted from pleading with God to come to his rescue. I can't help but relate to verse 8:

Has God forgotten to be gracious? Has he slammed the door on his compassion? And I said, "This is my fate; the Most High has turned his hand against me."

David's transparency and humanity in this passage gave me permission to feel the same way and approach God in the same way. I wondered when God might come to my rescue or if He was hearing my prayers at all.

THE BOTTOM

Welcome to the bottom of my pit. It's dark here. Hope seems distant and mocking. I'm trying to believe that I will be released from this pain and feel happy again. I'm not sure how. I am torn between obligations with work, house chores, church, and other obligations and desperately wanting, needing to isolate myself so I can give myself permission to be sad for a while—a long while. During my commute to work, I fantasize about getting in a car accident resulting in minor injuries that would require a short-term stay in the hospital where I could be completely removed from all obligations and responsibilities for a while. My friends, if you can relate to thinking like this, it's your mind and body trying to get your attention saying, "Hey, something is way out of balance right now. Self-care needed. Stop ignoring the problem. Address the wound and take time to heal."

I would love to think that I was self-aware enough to say that I recognized all this as a warning sign, but nope. I carried on feeling more and more weight on my shoulders. I knew that Matthew 11:28 said, *"Come to me, all you who are weary and burdened, and I will give you rest."* (NIV) But I wasn't sure if rest was even possible for me. I had been figuratively and literally holding my breath for years—ten years to be exact. Holding it together and suppressing my every emotion was the only way to get by. My threshold for pushing down all my emotions used to be a lot stronger, but not anymore. I was barely holding it together. Years of practice helped me to perfect small talk and smiles without anyone ever getting a glimpse of the dam of pain I was holding back.

> Journal Entries from March 28, 2016:
>
> *Do you not know? Have you not heard? The LORD is the everlasting God, the Creator of the ends of the earth. He will not grow tired or weary, and his understanding no one can fathom.*
>
> – Isaiah 40:28 NIV
>
> I have been afraid to journal. I am so angry on the inside, but I also don't know how to feel. I'm not sure how to process the information that my genetics are working against me to produce life. This is something I can't fix. I have no control. I am disappointed and frustrated.

> Journal Entries from April 15, 2016:
>
> I've been resonating with the song "What I know" by Tricia Brock on her Radiate album: It's such a good reminder that no matter what happens or how I feel, God never changes. He is always there.
>
> God, I trust Your goodness and rely on Your faithfulness. I hear You drawing me out encouraging me to hold onto hope. Help me to see Your purpose in all of this. What is the message You want me to share?

> Journal Entries from April 17, 2016:
>
> I am learning what it means to praise You in the midst of loss. There is a deep surrender that occurs with praising when it makes no sense. I have no control over my circumstances. I can't change it, so I'm left with frustration, anger, questions, and helplessness; then I find myself surrendering it all in a moment of worship, and my heart becomes unburdened.
>
> *Give your burdens to the LORD, and he will take care of you. He will not permit the godly to slip and fall.*
>
> – Psalm 55:22

What is the price of two sparrows—one copper coin? But not a single sparrow can fall to the ground without your Father knowing it. And the very hairs on your head are all numbered. So don't be afraid; you are more valuable to God than a whole flock of sparrows.

– Matthew 10:29–31

Then Jesus said, "Come to me, all of you who are weary and carry heavy burdens, and I will give you rest. Take my yoke upon you. Let me teach you, because I am humble and gentle, and you will find rest for your souls.

For my yoke is easy to bear, and the burden I give you is light."

– Matthew 11:28–30

Blessed is the one who perseveres under trial because, having stood the test, that person will receive the crown of life that the Lord has promised to those who love him.

– James 1:12 NIV (emphasis added)

- Persevere – under misfortunes and trials to hold fast to one's faith in Christ. To endure, bear bravely and calmly.
- The crown – a mark of royal or exalted rank; a wreath or garland given as a prize to victors; eternal blessedness; an ornament of honor.
- Of life – the state of one who possesses vitality; fullness of life belonging to God; devoted to God; blessed in this world as one who puts their trust in God.

Journal Entries from May 15, 2016:

I am learning the secret to overcoming the deep, indescribable pain that comes from loss and grief: praise. True surrender comes through praise. Burdens are lifted through praise.

Praise the LORD! Praise the LORD from the heavens! Praise Him from the skies!

– Psalm 148:1

Let all that I am praise the LORD; with my whole heart, I will praise his holy name.

– Psalm 103:1

But I will keep on hoping for your help; I will praise you more and more.

– Psalm 71:14

Praise the LORD; praise God our Savior! For each day he carries us in his arms.

– Psalm 68:19

Let all that I am praise the LORD; may I never forget the good things he does for me.

– Psalm 103:2

Praise the LORD! How good to sing praises to our God! How delightful and how fitting!

– Psalm 147:1

I will praise you, LORD, with all my heart; I will tell of all the marvelous things you have done

– Psalm 9:1

I will praise you as long as I live, lifting up my hands to you in prayer.

–Psalm 63:4

Why am I discouraged? Why is my heart so sad? I will put my hope in God! I will praise him again—my Savior and my God!

– Psalm 42:56a

But each day the Lord pours his unfailing love upon me, and through each night I sing his songs, praying to God who gives me life.

– Psalm 42:8

Even when everything is working against me to produce life, God gives me life. His love is unfailing, unrelenting. Thank You, Jesus, for pouring out Your love. I praise You!

Journal Entries from June 28, 2016:

I am weary from grief. It weighs so heavy on me. God, do You see my pain? Have You left me? Have I messed up or failed You? Is this Your purpose for me? I have lost my vision. I am so heartbroken! Please help me. Carry me. Hold me. I give up. I surrender. I don't know what else to do. Everyone keeps singing my praises telling me how strong I am—how amazed they are that I could go through so much loss and still trust in Your promises. The thing is that trusting You is not the hard part. I am still left with all this heartache, pain, loss, grief. I don't know what to do with that. While I trust You and believe that You're good, I am still really mad at You. I want to scream and yell and ask why You haven't come to my rescue. Why does it feel like You've abandoned me? Step in and do something! Meet me halfway. Do something.

> With all the stress of life as of late, my panic attacks have hit an all-time high. I let work know that I would need to work remotely for the month of June while I worked on healing. So in a very short time, we learned we can't have kids in the traditional method; Flip got laid off; we had to move and buy a new car; we had no hot water where we were living; and I continued to struggle with panic attacks. It all just felt like too much to handle all at once. I asked work if I could take unpaid leave for about ten days to get away and hit the reset button. They were nothing but supportive.

My emotional reserve was holding on by a thread—a very weak, fragile thread. Flip had just moved us into our new apartment, and I still had a week off from work. I dedicated my remaining days to focus on healing. I had to. I read through two books: Get Out of that Pit by Beth Moore and Coming Clean by Seth Haines. I needed to get out of my own head and get some fresh perspective. The new apartment community had a lovely pool area with palm trees, private cabanas, and a side courtyard with a Spanish-tiled gas fireplace. Every morning that week, I planted myself at a table near the fireplace with a view of the palm trees and pool. I brought my iced vanilla latte along with my books, my Bible, and my journal. I was not leaving until I had answers. At the very least, I finally had the time to vent and get it all out. This was between God and me.

> Journal Entries from June 30, 2016:
>
> I'm not fond of silence. Silence in the Bible is compared to death—"silent as the grave." I think of no heartbeat, no breath, no life. Silence is a scary place—a place of isolation. In a vision a few years back, I saw ten people on fire. They were screaming in pain, but no sound could be heard. They didn't even have the relief of expressing their pain. It was sheer torment. But I wonder if I've had a small dose of the same torment, not being able to express my pain. In a sense, I've been screaming, and no one has heard me. I've been slowly dying on the inside. I've been afraid to touch those wounded spots because they've gotten so much worse over time. Holy Spirit, You are the healer and comforter. There is nothing I can do. Please heal me and bring fresh life and revelation into this pain.
>
> I'm not a fan of silence. Silence is what happens when toddlers are getting into trouble. Silence is what occurs right before the principal can see you. Silence is where fear and darkness live. Yet apparently, healing and truth can be found in silence as well.
>
> What am I afraid of?
>
> - Death

- Loss
- Pain
- Rejection

Each time he said, "My grace is all you need. My power works best in weakness." So now I am glad to boast about my weaknesses, so that the power of Christ can work through me. That's why I take pleasure in my weaknesses, and in the insults, hardships, persecutions, and troubles that I suffer for Christ. For when I am weak, then I am strong.

– 2 Corinthians 12:9–10

I read these verses, and I envy Paul's perspective. I wonder what revelation he received that allowed him to be so content with such circumstances. I need to stop drowning my anxieties and start taking note of them.

Journal Entries from July 1, 2016:

Yesterday, I watched a bee climb to the top of a thin pane of glass separating the patio from the community pool. The bee slipped off the top of the pane of glass and struggled to regain its footing. I could see its legs kicking and trying to regain footing on top of the glass. I wanted to help somehow, but there's no way I was going to get close to the stinger. I felt anxiety and panic on behalf of the bee at the thought of how far it could fall. He struggled for what felt like forever. I asked God to please extend mercy and to relieve my anxiety watching the struggle. The bee continued to kick its legs. Then suddenly in an instant, it flew away.

I just sat there in astonishment and half laughed. The bee was capable of saving himself the entire time. The struggle was for nothing. I felt the Holy Spirit impress upon me that I too have the ability to "fly" away—that I have wings to save myself. I thought about this all day and all night. What do I have that can save me? At about four in the morning, it dawned on me. I have Scripture. I have the powerful word of God to fight, and I haven't been using it. I have been feeling isolated, hopeless, defenseless because I haven't been using the greatest weapon I have—my sword—the truth. No more lies. No more self-pity. No more self-loathing. Please God, forgive me for turning away from You when I should have turned into You as my hope and comfort. Forgive me for entertaining lies instead of listening to Your truth—truth about who I am and the future You've written for me from the beginning. Thank You for never leaving me—even in those moments when I was convinced that I was sitting in the darkness of my pit by myself.

Beth Moore says that "One of the biggest mistakes we could ever make is to assume that passionate desire is wrong, and that the goal for godly people is to not feel."[21]

Journal Entries from July 5, 2016:

Good morning, Lord. Everything goes back to the usual routine starting Friday. I'm nervous about connecting with everyone at work again. But I love my team, and I know they've got my back.

> *Watch this: God's eye is on those who respect him, the ones who are looking for his love. He's ready to come to their rescue in bad times; in lean times he keeps body and soul together. We're depending on GOD; he's everything we need. What's more, our hearts brim with joy since we've taken for our own his holy name. Love us, GOD, with all you've got—that's what we're depending on.*
>
> – Psalm 33:18–22 MSG

I had a dream the other night that I heard construction noise. I looked up and saw scaffolding on the moon. I asked God, "What is this?" He said, "I'm building you the moon, so your eyes won't hurt when I shine light on the dark places."

Several thoughts occur to me. God cares so much about my pain and healing that He'd build me the moon to ease the process as He lets the light (truth) of His Son reflect on the dark places of my soul. He loves me and is very present during this season.

God, thank You for taking me through this process of healing slowly. I have been afraid that removing one stone might cause the whole dam to crumble and drown me in my sorrows. Thank You for being so patient with me.

My mind is flooded with so many questions...

- Will we still have kids naturally?
- If we try, will we lose more babies to miscarriage?
- Are we being reckless to try again naturally apart from IVF or adoption?
- Is IVF still an option even though it costs so much?
- I believe we will adopt, but should we start the process now?

It's confusing to have options at all. My brain saw this whole process of having children as being so simple... and it's not. I think I might be ready. God, can You shed some light on one of the dark places in my heart?

The dark place is uncertainty. I don't have answers for the pain. Why did we lose five babies? God is sovereign. He sees all things. He created all things. God is good and faithful and loves me. Then why allow such heartache and pain? Why give me a promise that I will have a home and become a happy mother only to have two more miscarriages and receive news of a genetic condition called chromosomal translocation? I try to rationalize and reconcile my faith, God's goodness, God's will, and the deep tragedies of life. I cannot explain it all away. It makes no sense. I didn't deserve it or bring it on myself. I'm not sure my level of faith or the number of prayers could have made a difference at all. I'm left to wonder why God didn't intervene on my behalf. Why didn't He come to my rescue or protect me? I have been abandoned.

This is definitely a dark place I have hidden. How can I call myself a Christian when I am doubting that God can be trusted? I write out the truths of Scripture. I remind myself of times of answered prayers—times when I've clearly heard the voice of God directing my life. I muster just enough hope to give me the courage to face another day. Am I a fraud? Do I masquerade as a faith-filled believer when secretly my soul is screaming, "God has left me!" I cannot reconcile the mystery of God or His will. I am left only with the option of surrender.

In Matthew 26:42, Jesus surrendered to the pain and torture of crucifixion, separation from God, and the excruciating weight of the sin of the world. He accepted it all as the will of God, and in turn, salvation was made available to all mankind. Relationship with God, the Father, was restored.

> *Father, if you are willing, take this cup away from me; yet not my will, but yours, be done.*
>
> – Luke 22:42 NIV

Journal Entries from July 10, 2016:

Characteristics of a pit:

- You feel stuck.
- You can't stand up.
- You've lost your vision.

Waiting patiently for the Lord is not about doing nothing to be rescued. It's about posturing yourself in absolute expectation.

God has already given His word to provide us with a home and cause me to become a joyous mother. In Psalm 113:9, I already have His "Yes." So, it's not a matter of yes or no. It's a matter of living with great expectation in how this will be accomplished. I'm not going to hold anything back anymore. Whether we have a natural birth, IVF, or adoption, I will be a happy mother. I long to pour life into my babies, to nurture them and encourage them to try everything and run hard after their dreams.

> *But blessed are those who trust in the LORD and have made the LORD their hope and confidence.*
>
> –Jeremiah 17:7

Isaiah 43:1–2, 5–6, 13, 18–19:

> *Do not be afraid, for I have ransomed you. I have called you by name; you are mine. When you go through deep waters and great trouble, I will be with you. When you go through rivers of difficulty, you will not drown! When you walk through the fire of oppression, you will not be burned up; the flames will not consume you... Do not be afraid, for I am with you. I will gather you and your children from east and west and from north and south... From eternity to eternity I am God. No one can snatch anyone out of my hand. No one can undo what I have done... But forget all that —it is nothing compared to what I am going to do. For I am about to do something new. See, I have already begun! Do you not see it? I will make a pathway through the wilderness. I will create rivers in the dry wasteland.*

Only God can create something from nothing. I trust You with my fears and with my doubts and uncertainties. I trust You with my life and the lives of my babies. My future is in Your hands. I cling to You with stubborn expectation that You will honor Your promises while I yet breathe. Thank You for loving me.

These are the biggest revelations that came out of this time of reading, venting, and journaling:

- I'm not powerless in my despair. I have a powerful weapon I have not been taking advantage of—Scripture.
- God cares about my healing process. He is protective of my heart.
- Surrender means trusting God with my future even when I don't have any answers.

Lifelines

QUESTIONS TO CONSIDER

What revelations is God showing you in the midst of your healing journey?

How is your perspective shifting?

Where is your focus?

SCRIPTURE VERSES

I waited patiently for the LORD; he turned to me and heard my cry. He lifted me out of the slimy pit, out of the mud and mire; he set my feet on a rock and gave me a firm place to stand. He put a new song in my mouth, a hymn of praise to our God. Many will see and fear the LORD and put their trust in him. – Psalm 40:1–3 NIV

David crying to God for help in Psalm 77:1–12

Why am I discouraged? Why is my heart so sad? I will put my hope in God! I will praise Him again—my Savior and my God! – Psalm 42:5–6a

Hope deferred makes the heart sick, but a dream fulfilled is a tree of life.
– Proverbs 13:12

WORSHIP SONGS

"Out of Hiding" by Steffany Gretzinger from her *The Undoing* album.

"Open up Let the Light In" by Steffany Gretziniger from her *The Undoing* album.

Bethel Worship. "I Am No Victim" by Bethel Worship from the *Where His Light Was* album.

"God That Saves" (feat. Stephen McWhirter) by Iron Bell Music from the *God That Saves* album.

"Jireh" (feat. Chandler Moore & Naomi Raine) by Elevation Worship, Maverick City Music.

"Don't You Give Up On Me" by Brandon Lake from the *HELP!* album.

SERMONS

"How to Deal with Dark Times" by Tim Keller[22]

QUOTES

God's timing is designed to teach us to trust. It's not designed to give us relief. It's designed to give us revelation." - Steven Furtick[23]

"You face your greatest opposition when you're closest to your biggest miracle." - T. D. Jakes[24]

"Stop watering things that were never meant to grow in your life. Water what works, what's good, what's right. Stop playing around with those dead bones and stuff you can't fix, it's over…leave it alone! You're coming into a season of greatness. If you water what's alive and divine, you will see harvest like you've never seen before." - T. D. Jakes[25]

BOOKS

Coming Clean by Seth Haines.

Get Out of That Pit by Beth Moore.

PRAYER

God, there is nothing left to do but surrender. My life is Yours. Take these broken pieces and mend this heart. I trust You with my future. I relinquish the expectations I've been holding fast to in regard to the future I was planning for myself. Show me what You have in store. I am still clinging to the promise You gave me. Thank You for Your faithfulness despite my fears and persistent doubts. Please continue to be patient with me as You help me to navigate my way through this dark season one step at a time. In Jesus' name, Amen.

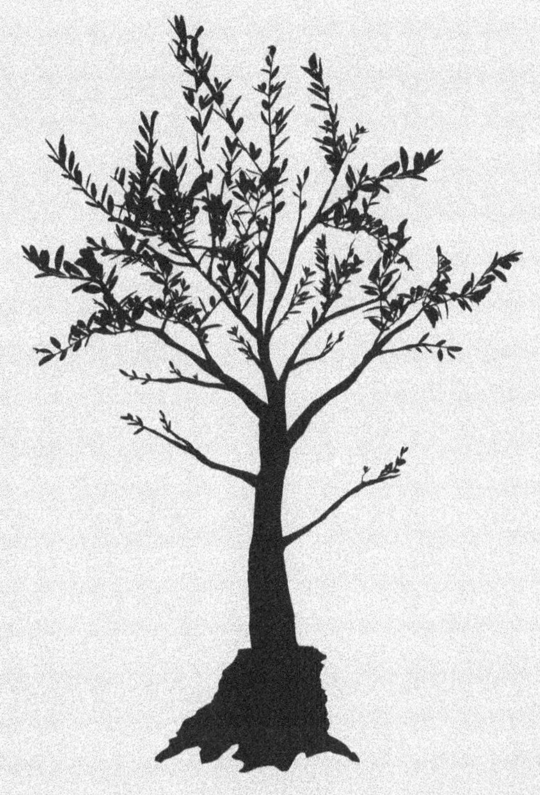

GOD SAID... *lead with praise.*

Jericho

He gives the barren woman a home, so that she becomes a happy mother. Praise the LORD! – Psalm 113:9

IN THE BIBLE, GOD'S CHOSEN PEOPLE, THE ISRAELITES, WERE RESCUED FROM SLAVERY in Egypt by Aaron and Moses. You may have heard the story of Pharaoh and the ten plagues. Somewhere between 2 and 3 million Israelite men, women, and children were led out of Egypt and into the wilderness. God was visible to His people as a pillar of cloud by day and a pillar of fire by night. It must have been nice to have that physical assurance of the God's presence leading their way. Incredible miracles took place with the parting of the Red Sea, bread (manna) from heaven, water from rocks, and more. God's provision for His people came through the miraculous. The Israelites finally had an opportunity to take possession of the land God had promised them—the Promised Land—but fear of the giants in the land prevented them from taking action. For this reason, they ended up wandering through the wilderness for forty years until Joshua led the people into the Promised Land. The very first victory for the Israelites in the Promised Land was the city of Jericho.

Joshua 6:1–5, 8–17, 20:

> *Now the gates of Jericho were tightly shut because the people were afraid of the Israelites. No one was allowed to go out or in. But the LORD said to Joshua, "I have given you Jericho, its king, and all its strong warriors. You and your fighting men should march around the town once a day for six days. Seven priests will walk ahead of the Ark, each carrying a ram's horn. On the seventh day you are to march around the town seven times, with the priests blowing the horns. When you hear the priests give one long blast on the rams' horns, have all the people shout as loud as they can. Then the*

walls of the town will collapse, and the people can charge straight into the town...

After Joshua spoke to the people, the seven priests with the rams' horns started marching in the presence of the LORD, blowing the horns as they marched. And the Ark of the LORD's Covenant followed behind them. Some of the armed men marched in front of the priests with the horns and some behind the Ark, with the priests continually blowing the horns. "Do not shout; do not even talk," Joshua commanded. "Not a single word from any of you until I tell you to shout. Then shout!" So the Ark of the LORD was carried around the town once that day, and then everyone returned to spend the night in the camp.

Joshua got up early the next morning, and the priests again carried the Ark of the LORD. The seven priests with the rams' horns marched in front of the Ark of the LORD, blowing their horns. Again the armed men marched both in front of the priests with the horns and behind the Ark of the LORD. All this time the priests were blowing their horns. On the second day they again marched around the town once and returned to the camp. They followed this pattern for six days.

On the seventh day the Israelites got up at dawn and marched around the town as they had done before. But this time they went around the town seven times. The seventh time around, as the priests sounded the long blast on their horns, Joshua commanded the people, "Shout! For the LORD has given you the town! Jericho and everything in it must be completely destroyed as an offering to the LORD"... When the people heard the sound of the rams' horns, they shouted as loud as they could. Suddenly, the walls of Jericho collapsed, and the Israelites charged straight into the town and captured it.

I don't know if I'm the only one who has this reaction, but doesn't this story seem absolutely crazy? The Israelites must have thought that Joshua had completely lost his mind. How in the world is marching around the walls of Jericho going to give us victory? It doesn't make any sense. So, we're supposed to march around the city walls just one time for six days straight and not say a word. And then on the seventh day, we march around seven times and shout and declare that the Lord has given us victory over Jericho. And that's it? Uh-huh.

Oftentimes, trusting in God looks exactly like this. God gave me a promise that I would have a home and become a happy mother in the same way that He declared the Israelites would have victory over the city of Jericho. We continued to try getting pregnant naturally even though past experience and doctors were telling us our chances were not good. It didn't make sense to keep trying, but we did it anyway and approached each pregnancy choosing to celebrate those little lives for as long as we had them.

If marching around the walls seven times brought victory into God's promises for the Israelites, this is what the seventh time around looked like for us.

> Journal Entry from September 11, 2016:
>
> I'm not even sure where to begin. My thoughts are overwhelmed. I have been longing for a few minutes (hours) to log my thoughts—get it all out. On August 23rd, I took a pregnancy test on a whim, and sure enough... positive! We decided to reserve the news for a few friends we knew would partner and fight with us in prayer. I'm about six weeks along at this point; historically, this is when we would be seeing signs of loss, such as cramping, fading symptoms, and bleeding. Instead, I'm experiencing morning (all day) sickness for the first time. We are both very encouraged and daring to hope for more this time around. It's as if I can practically taste everything. Laundry detergent, deodorant, eucalyptus trees—everything smells so strong. I have to eat every two hours, or the nausea comes back. I was telling my dearest friend how miserably grateful I am. I took a blood test this last Thursday morning, and I will have another blood test tomorrow morning to check HCG levels. I am holding out hope that I will get to hold this beautiful baby. I am overwhelmed with joy and keep telling myself to focus on God's promise and not let fear creep in. It would be so easy to entertain thoughts of dread, grief, and loss and to allow myself to expect the worst. And why not—history has not given me anything else. But I can't go there. I can't live in fear. I love this little life and choose to keep my focus on this:
>
> > *You made all the delicate inner parts of my body and knit me together in my mother's womb. Thank you for making me so wonderfully complex! Your workmanship is marvelous—how well I know it.*
> >
> > – Psalm 139:13–14
>
> This baby is being knit together by the hand of God. I am so blessed to be a part of His marvelous workmanship.
>
> I had a great moment this last week. I bought some frozen pot stickers because I had a craving. I cooked half the bag and put the rest away. When I decided I wanted to cook a few more, I couldn't find them anywhere. I looked in the freezer, the fridge, the plate cupboard—no dice. I felt like I was losing my mind. I couldn't figure out where in the world they could have disappeared to. Then I opened the pantry, and there they were next to the cans of soup! I laughed so hard. It was official—pregnancy brain is

real. Haha!

Journal Entry from September 14, 2016:

One moment, I am overjoyed and full of hope. The next moment, I am filled with fear and worry wondering if today is the day that I'll start bleeding. I want this baby so badly, and all I can do is surrender and remind myself that God's promises are true. He can be trusted to keep His word. Everything is out of my control. It's difficult at times to lean into Him when I feel like flailing. I received amazing news yesterday that my HCG levels are rising. Thank you, Jesus!

A few hours later, I got a call from the pharmacy saying Dr. Cortez ordered me progesterone. I haven't talked to Dr. Cortez. I don't know if this is preventative or necessary. My joy went straight to concern. I desperately wish I could do more to ensure that the baby will be okay. Close friends at church keep praying for a healthy, whole baby—full of life and thriving! My heart echoes those prayers as well.

Dear God, please continue to knit this little one together into Your wonderful workmanship. Please provide me with an extra dose of courage today. Help me to fall back into surrender and let this fear and worry wash away. Thank You for holding all of us in Your hands. Thank You for knowing me so well.

Journal Entry from September 15, 2016:

Today, I woke up full of hope. I have a beautiful life growing inside of me. I wondered if it would even be possible without help. God, my heart is so full of gratitude. Thank You for blessing me with life. Continue to knit this little one with Your hands. This baby is such a beacon of hope and light.

> *But let the godly rejoice. Let them be glad in God's presence. Let them be filled with joy.*
>
> – Psalm 68:3

Journal Entry from October 3, 2016:

In the last month and a half, I have been feeling a constant state of nausea. Glorious nausea confirming that hormones are surging and baby is alive and thriving. We had our first ultrasound last Monday. Admittedly, my heart was in my throat, and I braced myself for the worst possible news. I expected to hear, "Don't worry. You're really early. It's normal to not see the heartbeat yet. We'll try again at your next appointment." Flip and I gripped each other's hands as the nurse announced within two seconds, "Oh! There's the heartbeat!" We both melted instantly and cried and laughed with joy. We saw the heartbeat and baby's little arms and legs move around. It was the most amazing, breathtaking experience. Pure joy and relief! We were so overjoyed that I took the day off work! We had to celebrate! We called friends and family and cried more tears of joy! We spent the day glowing and celebrated with good food and the new movie Storks. It was such a perfect day!

> *For the LORD is good. His unfailing love continues forever, and his faithfulness continues to each generation.*
>
> – Psalm 100:5

> *You satisfy me more than the richest feast. I will praise you with songs of joy.*
>
> – Psalm 63:5

Journal Entry from January 2, 2017:

I am overwhelmed by Your blessings and Your faithfulness. You are the God of miracles. You are so good. Thank You for keeping Your promises.

> *For I am about to do something new. See, I have already begun! Do you not see it? I will make a pathway through the wilderness. I will create rivers in the dry wasteland.*
>
> – Isaiah 43:19

Only You, God, can create life from nothing and make a way where there is no way. As of yesterday, we are six months pregnant. It still seems so unreal to even say. I am in awe of where we are right now. I am so grateful to have this experience. I have felt the baby move. Others have described it as a fluttering, but it actually feels kinda like my stomach grumbling, but in places where my stomach isn't. It's so fun. The due date is April 23rd, so we have less than four months to go. It's going by so fast. I'm so proud of our little one and how strong baby is getting. We find out the gender in two weeks. Our friends are throwing us a gender reveal party, and we're hosting it at the clubhouse at our place. I'm nervous and excited. Discovering the gender will be one step closer to getting to know our little one. Part of me feels a little emotionally disconnected, but I think it's because we've never gotten this far before. We have only had bad news before now. And now everything is suddenly by the book and perfect.

> *Remember your promise to me; it is my only hope. Your promise revives*

me; it comforts me in all my troubles.

– Psalm 119:49–50

Your word is everything to me. It is my lifeline. I trust You with my whole heart and with the lives of those I love and hold close. Thank You for loving me so deeply and being so gentle with my broken heart. Your love has healed those places where I thought I could never feel again. Thank You for the honor of becoming a mother. Thank You for the friends and church family who have surrounded us with love.

He gives the barren woman a home, so that she becomes a happy mother. Praise the LORD!

– Psalm 113:9

I feel honored to be among the ranks of Hannah, Sarah, Rachel, and all the other women of the faith who have gone before me trusting God with their futures and ability to produce life.

I will praise the LORD at all times. I will constantly speak his praises. I will boast only in the LORD; let all who are take heart. Come, let us tell of the LORD's greatness; let us exalt his name together. I prayed to the LORD, and he answered me, freeing me from all my fears.

– Psalm 34:1–4

Journal Entry from January 8, 2017:

Good morning, Lord. Happy Sunday! I continue to feel beyond blessed. Baby is 25 weeks old today. I feel more and more movement every day. It's quite miraculous, and I feel fortunate to experience every moment. Flip got to feel the baby move for the first time yesterday. It completely filled my heart with joy.

I echo the sentiment expressed by Chris Tomlin: "Worship isn't something we do out of obligation, but rather in response to who God is and what He has done."[26] I am in awe of Your goodness.

Journal Entry from January 22, 2017:

God, I am so in awe of Your goodness! We are having a little boy! I can hardly believe it. Thank You for answered prayers and kept promises. I am so honored to be a part of this journey You have us on. Parenthood is three months away. My heart is so full of joy! Thank You for pouring your blessings on us.

> *You thrill me, LORD, with all you have done for me! I sing for joy because of what you have done. O LORD, what great miracles you do! And how deep are your thoughts.*
>
> – Psalm 92:4–5
>
> *He will cover you with his feathers. He will shelter you with his wings. His faithful promises are your armor and protection.*
>
> – Psalm 91:4

Flip and I could not for the life of us agree on a name for our little guy. We went back and forth on a few options, but none of them felt like "the one." It was also scary determining a permanent name for our little person. Choosing someone's name is not only an honor as a parent but a terrifying responsibility. We had to consider what kinds of names kids in school would use as nicknames, or if the name we chose would encourage a lifetime of teasing and torture. We decided to spend a week praying and seeking God separately about the name that would fit him best. After a week passed, we met and both of us shared the same name: Jericho. It's a very uncommon name, and we both felt confident with God's leading on it, especially in light of the story of Jericho in the Bible. As we read the story earlier, the city of Jericho was the Israelites' first victory in God's promised land. The Israelites walked around the city walls first for six days led by worshipers with horns. Walking around the walls of a city didn't make any sense, but they obeyed. On the seventh day marching around the city, they gave a shout, and the walls of Jericho fell, and the victory was theirs!

This echoed our story in so many ways. We experienced six losses prior to Jericho, but we chose to worship God and celebrate every single life for however long we were blessed to have them. It must have seemed crazy for the Israelites to walk around the city walls of Jericho for six days expecting those walls to somehow come crumbling down. In the same way, it may have seemed absolutely crazy for us to keep trying to have a baby. Why risk more loss, devastation, grief, and heartache? But we chose to surrender and worship no matter the outcome. Jericho was our seventh pregnancy and the fulfillment of God's promise to us.

He gives the barren woman a home, so that she becomes a happy mother. Praise the LORD!

– Psalm 113:9

> Journal entry from February 19, 2017:
>
> God, I am continually blown away at Your goodness. We do not have any of the essentials (in my opinion) ready for our baby boy. We have a few

diapers and onesies but no crib, stroller, or other essentials. I have been wondering how we would be able to save for these items costing nearly $1,000 in total. Our family came to visit yesterday and took us shopping for a top-of-the-line stroller plus accessories. We were so blessed by their generosity! They also gave us cash to order the crib online and buy a new infant car seat!

God, You are so good! Thank You for meeting these needs and helping my heart and nerves to be at peace and rest for the arrival of our son. I am feeling so much more prepared.

> *You will keep in perfect peace all who trust in you, all whose thoughts are fixed on you! Trust in the LORD always, for the LORD GOD is the eternal Rock.*
>
> – Isaiah 26:3–4

Journal Entry from March 8, 2017:

God, I am in awe of the outpouring of blessing in our lives right now. We decided on the name Jericho Dale Flippin. The city of Jericho was the first Israelite victory in the promised land. And that's exactly how we feel about our little man.

Good friends of ours paid for us to attend Nicole Green's birthing classes. We had our first class last Wednesday. Nicole is amazing! These classes typically last ten weeks and cost $495. It was a huge and generous gift.

Our church is throwing us a co-ed baby shower this Saturday, March 11th. I'm really looking forward to it—especially the prayer time. The games look to be hilarious!

I'm thirty-three weeks pregnant now. Only seven weeks until we get to meet Jericho and see his miraculous face. We have never come this far before, and I find myself a little anxious about labor and delivery. Nicole's birthing classes will definitely help with being mentally prepared and bring more peace of mind about the process. I seriously can't believe what my body is capable of. I have heard horror stories, and then I also hear how moms would do it all over again. My body is definitely not my own right now. It is difficult to find a comfortable position to sleep in, and there are fun things like heartburn and leg cramps at this stage. But these are such minor inconveniences for the privilege of bearing life. The whole process is so mind-blowing. Thank You, God, that we get to experience this version of Your creation. So beautiful and terrifying and glorious!

How great is the goodness you have stored up for those who fear you. You lavish it on those who come to you for protection, blessing them before the watching world.

– Psalm 31:19

The LORD is good, a strong refuge when trouble comes. He is close to those who trust in him.

– Nahum 1:7

He gives the barren woman a home, so that she becomes a happy mother. Praise the LORD!

– Psalm 113:9

He will cover you with his feathers. He will shelter you with his wings. His faithful promises are your armor and protection.

– Psalm 91:4

Journal Entry from May 10, 2017:

I can relate to Mary in a small way when it says in Luke 2:19 that Mary quietly treasured (or pondered) these things in her heart and thought about them often. I am so beyond blessed to have our sweet baby in our arms. My water broke at six thirty Saturday morning, April 22nd. Labor and contractions started around eight o'clock that morning. We transitioned from home to the hospital at nine o'clock that evening when the contractions felt like they were building momentum. I thought waiting until nine o'clock was a decent amount of time to labor at home in hopes that I would be closer to delivery by the time we arrived at the hospital. Turns out, I was only three centimeters dilated upon arrival to the hospital, but I was still hopeful to meet our little man by morning on his actual due date of April 23rd. Leave it to Jericho to beat the odds and be one of the three percent of babies born on their actual due date.

However, he was not born by the morning. I had labored all day and all night, and I was only 6.5 centimeters dilated. While the amazing nurses on duty were praising my progress, I wanted to cry at the slow progress. We passed the 24-hour mark from the time my water broke. Normally, they would insist on induction to avoid the risk of infection, but they allowed me to keep laboring because Jericho and I were still going strong—no issues with heart rate, blood pressure, or fever. At the 30-hour mark, my contractions were getting further apart—with eleven minutes between each one. Alison (our midwife) recommended Pitocin to get Jericho born faster. I was exhausted and didn't want to experience Pitocin on an empty tank, so I asked if it was too late to introduce an epidural before they started the Pitocin. They said that was no problem. So, we prepared for both. These measures were obviously straying from our birth preferences, and Flip was not thrilled about feeling like I was "off limits" with all the tubes and wires I was connected to. But at the same time, we felt confident in the decisions being made because of all the preparations we received in Nicole's birthing classes. After four more hours and increasing Pitocin over five times, I was only at 8.5–9 centimeters dilated. We decided to start pushing to encourage my body to reach 10 centimeters. Pushing normally only takes a max of three hours, but after four hours, Jericho's poor little head was getting swollen from hitting my tailbone with every contraction.

Things were taking too long, and both Jericho and I started to run a slight fever. They brought in Dr. Lopez, the on-call doctor. She let us know that time was running out, and we had three tries with the vacuum to try to get Jericho out; if not, they would have to do a cesarean section. I was adamantly opposed to cesarean with Jericho being so close. The vacuum didn't suction on the first try. It briefly suctioned on the second try, but no luck. On the third try, it didn't seem like the vacuum was going to work (and it didn't), so I pushed harder than ever. On my last breath with the contraction, Jericho's head came, and then his body emerged. He was crying, and it was the most beautiful thing I've ever heard! One breath away from a c-section and after thirty-eight hours, Jericho Dale Flippin was born at 7:58 p.m. on April 23, 2017. He weighed 8.5 pounds and measured 22 inches long. He'll be three weeks old on Sunday (Mother's Day), and I still can't believe he is ours. I am just in awe. So grateful to hold him and share life with this amazing person.

I will praise the LORD as long as I live. I will sing praises to my God with my dying breath.

– Psalm 146:2

He made heaven and earth, the sea, and everything in them. He keeps every promise forever.

– Psalm 146:6

JOY REBORN

Jericho showed me a depth of joy I didn't know was possible. You might be wondering if his miraculous entrance into our lives washed away eleven years of pain, loss, grief, and heartache. I wish it worked that way. I stepped into motherhood with both sheer joy for my son and continued great loss for my other sweet babies who didn't make it.

God absolutely knew what He was doing, and His timing could not have been better. After so many years of not allowing myself to feel anything, Jericho birthed in me a freedom to feel joy again. But with this fresh reawakening of my emotions to feel joy also came a sweeping wave of grief and heartache that I had been so diligent to ignore for years. I guess that old adage of "time heals all wounds" is a giant farse. Instead, I should have adopted this quote from The Princess Bride: "Life is pain, highness. Anyone who says differently is selling something."[27]

Over a series of quiet times with God, I felt Him nudge me and encourage me to embrace all my emotions again. This may sound sweet and simple, but I assure you my thoughts were screaming, "No way!! Uh-uh. Nope." I had worked hard over many years to shove those emotions deep, deep, deep, way deep down. And I still had that nagging inner voice telling me that I'd risk it all if I allowed myself to feel. People would think I was unhinged or too much to handle. However, I felt a gentle reassurance that I would not be alone in the process and that He would not allow me to drown in my sorrow like I was picturing in my head.

In this next season of healing, I discovered some amazing things. I thought Jericho was the fulfillment of God's promise in Psalm 113:9, but God didn't stop there. He was just getting started.

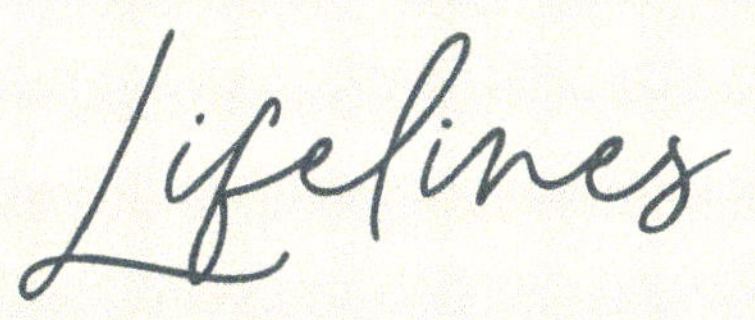

QUESTIONS TO CONSIDER

What does your fulfilled promise look like?

SCRIPTURE VERSES

He gives the barren woman a home, so that she becomes a happy mother. Praise the LORD!! – Psalm 113:9

You made all the delicate inner parts of my body and knit me together in my mother's womb. Thank you for making me so wonderfully complex! Your workmanship is marvelous —how well I know it. – Psalm 139:13–14

You will keep in perfect peace all who trust in you, all whose thoughts are fixed on you! Trust in the LORD always, for the LORD GOD is the eternal Rock. – Isaiah 26:3–4

For the LORD is good. His unfailing love continues forever, and his faithfulness continues to each generation. – Psalm 100:5

WORSHIP SONGS

"White Flag" by Fearless BND from the *We Are Fearless* album.

"Another in the Fire" by Hillsong UNITED from the *People (Live)* album.

Hillsong UNITED. "Oceans (Where Feet May Fail)" by Hillsong UNITED from the *Zion (Deluxe Edition)* album.

"Raise a Hallelujah" by Jonathan David Hesler and Melissa Hesler from *Raise a Hallelujah (Studio Version)*.

"See a Victory" by Elevation Worship from their *See a Victory* album.

"Promises" by Maverick City Music, Joe L Barnes, and Naomi Raine.

QUOTES

"You are not fighting for a victory... you're fighting from victory! Victory is already yours." - Priscilla Shirer[28]

PRAYER

God, Your goodness and faithfulness are beyond words! Thank You for answered prayer and fulfilled promises! I am in awe of Your good works. I praise You! Even in my deepest moments of heartache and doubt, You were still present and holding my hand through it all. Thank You for being a God of the impossible. Nothing is too hard for You. Thank You for loving me and blessing me with a promise come true!

part 2 | The Healing

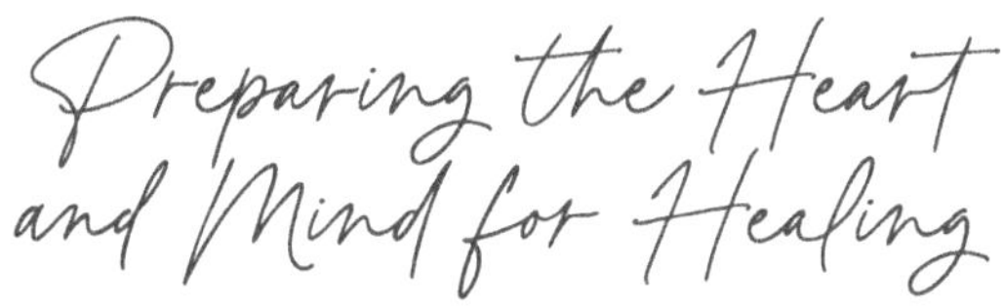

Before we dive into "Part 2: The Healing," it's important to set some expectations and clearly define what healing means. Prepare your heart and mind. Muster some of that well-earned grit from the experiences that life has handed you, roll up your sleeves, and let's look at what healing really means.

DEFINING KEY TERMS

heal (verb)

a. to make free from injury or disease: to make sound or whole.
b. to make well again: to restore to health.
c. to cause (an undesirable condition) to be overcome: MEND.
d. to patch up or correct (a breach or division).
e. to restore to original purity or integrity.[29]

health (noun)

a. the condition of being sound in body, mind, or spirit.
b. freedom from physical disease or pain.
c. the general condition of the body.
d. a condition in which someone or something is thriving or doing well: WELL-BEING.
e. general condition or state.[30]

restore (verb)

a. GIVE BACK, RETURN.
b. to put or bring back into existence or use.
c. to bring back to or put back into a former or original state: RENEW.
d. to put again in possession of something.[31]

renew (verb)

a. to make like new: restore to freshness, vigor, or perfection.
b. to make new spiritually: REGENERATE.
c. to restore to existence: REVIVE.
d. to make extensive changes in: REBUILD.
e. to do again: REPEAT.

f. to begin again: RESUME.
g. REPLACE, REPLENISH.[32]

thrive (verb)
a. to grow vigorously: FLOURISH.
b. to gain in wealth or possessions: PROSPER.
c. to progress toward or realize a goal despite or because of circumstances.[33]

flourish (verb)
a. to grow luxuriantly: THRIVE.
b. to achieve success: PROSPER.
c. to be in a state of activity or production.
d. to reach a height of development or influence.[34]

When taken together, the definitions for the words heal, health, restore, renew, thrive, and flourish make up a pattern of full restoration. A summary of the these definitions might look like this:

> Healing is freedom from pain, restoration of mind, body, and soul, and it facilitates growth toward a state of prosperity and influence.

God cares about healing and restoration. He would not have sent His only Son, Jesus, to die and take on all our pain if He didn't care.

> *For God so loved the world, that He gave His only Son, so that everyone who believes in Him will not perish, but have eternal life.*
>
> – John 3:16 NASB2020

> *After you have suffered for a little while, the God of all grace, who called you to His eternal glory in Christ, will Himself perfect, confirm, strengthen, and establish you.*
>
> – 1 Peter 5:10 NASB2020

> *He restores my soul; He guides me in the paths of righteousness for the sake of His name.*
>
> – Psalm 23:3 NASB2020

> *Restore our fortunes, LORD, as the streams in the South. Those who sow in tears shall harvest with joyful shouting.*
>
> – Psalm 126:4-5NASB2020

> *He heals the brokenhearted and binds up their wounds.*
>
> – Psalm 147:3 NASB2020

> *Heal me, LORD, and I will be healed; Save me and I will be saved, for You are my praise.*
>
> –Jeremiah 17:14 NASB2020

> *And He will wipe away every tear from their eyes; and there will no longer be any death; there will no longer be any mourning, or crying, or pain; the first things have passed away.*
>
> – Revelations 21:4 NASB2020

KEY EXPECTATIONS

With a better understanding of the concept of healing as outlined above, let's set some expectations on what the healing process looks like.

HEALING IS NOT INSTANTANEOUS

After suffering through tremendous pain and grief and trudging through the emotional, physical, and social repercussions from the losses I experienced, I was frustrated to learn that healing isn't instantaneous. After the torment of going through those experiences, it seemed only fair or even justified that the healing process should not be difficult or painful as well. Christine Caine references this reality in Unashamed:

> The pain of recovery can often be longer and more painful than the pain of the original wounding. It's not fair but it is reality. If you are willing to partner with Jesus, you will make it through to healing and wholeness. It's hard work, but noble work and worth it.[35]

Healing is a process. My mentor once described the healing process as a dead tree. In order to remove it safely, you have to cut down the branches before you can get to the trunk, and then you have to cut down sections of the trunk before you can pull out the stump and ultimately remove the roots.

Take a moment to acknowledge and set the expectation that healing is not instantaneous. The healing process may take a while. This time is incredibly valuable and precious. Don't rush it. Own it. Embrace it. Allow God to open your eyes and empower you with each step. You will gain so much more than you lost.

HEALING DOESN'T MEAN THAT YOU FORGET

I had the idea that being healed somehow meant that all the pain washed away as if it had never happened. What healing does is bring a shift in perspective that allows you to recall the event without being controlled by it any longer. Healing brings freedom. You don't forget, but you get to overcome. Take a moment to acknowledge and set this expectation.

HEALING REQUIRES HONESTY

Healing can't take place without honesty. When you've had pain for a long time, you become so familiar with it that it's easy to minimize it. Acknowledge the pain and the scope of the wound. Don't minimize, hide, or run from it. Talk through it with people you trust. Get mad. Find a safe place to process it completely. Don't ignore any piece of it; otherwise, it will fester and, like a physical wound, breed infection if not properly treated. Unhealed wounds breed anger, bitterness, isolation, and can ultimately result in physical symptoms, such as anxiety, depression, panic, or ulcers. The secret cure to approaching healing with honesty is the dreaded "f" word—forgiveness. Forgiveness is as vulnerable and honest as it gets. Forgiveness is the fastest path from wounded to warrior. I promise you'll be unstoppable on the other side of it.

HEALING TAKES TRUST

Trust is earned—even with God. When it comes to building trust, your relationship with God is like any other relationship. The more time you spend with God, the more you get to know Him. You'll go through experiences together and learn over time that God can be trusted. God has shown me in my weakest moments that I'm not alone. He hears me, He understands, and He can be trusted with my heart.

The trust part was the scariest step for me in my healing process. It took a long time for me to stop running from healing and trust God with the outcome. I had to surrender the life I expected to have. Too often, we have unrealistic social and cultural expectations that successful adulthood reflects all the same milestones for everyone. For instance, we may expect everyone's life to unfold the same: graduate from high school, attend college, acquire a good-paying job, meet your significant other, get married, buy a house, have a child, have more children, and so on. If you get stuck at any of these life milestones, you're tempted to feel the shame of failure. After Flip and I got married, I expected that we would have children eventually. With every loss, my sense of failure grew exponentially. Confronting my need for healing meant that I had to trust God with my future, even if it meant that we never had children or that our story might include struggle. The good news about surrendering to God is that He always fills the gap with so much more than what is released.

Healing takes trust; God can be trusted with your past, your present, and your future. Your heart and your story are in good hands.

> *Looking unto Jesus, the author and finisher of our faith, who for the joy that was set before Him endured the cross, despising the shame, and has sat down at the right hand of the throne of God.*
>
> – Hebrews 12:2 NKJV

> *For we are His workmanship, created in Christ Jesus for good works, which God prepared beforehand so that we would walk in them.*
>
> – Ephesians 2:10 NASB2020

KEY BENEFITS AND OUTCOMES

How do you know when healing has taken place? You'll be able to tell your story without the onslaught of emotions that formerly accompanied every memory. The healing process is something that no one asks for, but once you've gone through it, you gain a strength and resilience that no one can take from you.

BEFORE HEALING	AFTER HEALING
Heavy/Burdened	Light/Unburdened (Matthew 11:28–30)
Heartbroken	Comforted (2 Corinthians 1:3–4, Psalm 71:19–21)
Hopeless	Hopeful (Jeremiah 29:11)
Broken	Healed (Psalm 30:2)
Loss	Restoration (1 Peter 5:10, Psalm 126:5)

The healing process will look different for everyone. Thankfully, we have a God who knows us and knows what we need to walk through the pain.

> *Even though I walk through the valley of the shadow of death, I fear no evil, for You are with me; Your rod and Your staff, they comfort me.*
>
> – Psalm 23:4 NASB2020

The blessings that I experienced coming out of my pit caught me by surprise. I had lost so much, but God was faithful to restore above and beyond anything I could have imagined. I learned that I wasn't powerless and that I have superpowers readily available to slay the darkness. I'll share more about these superpowers in "Part 3: The Revelation."

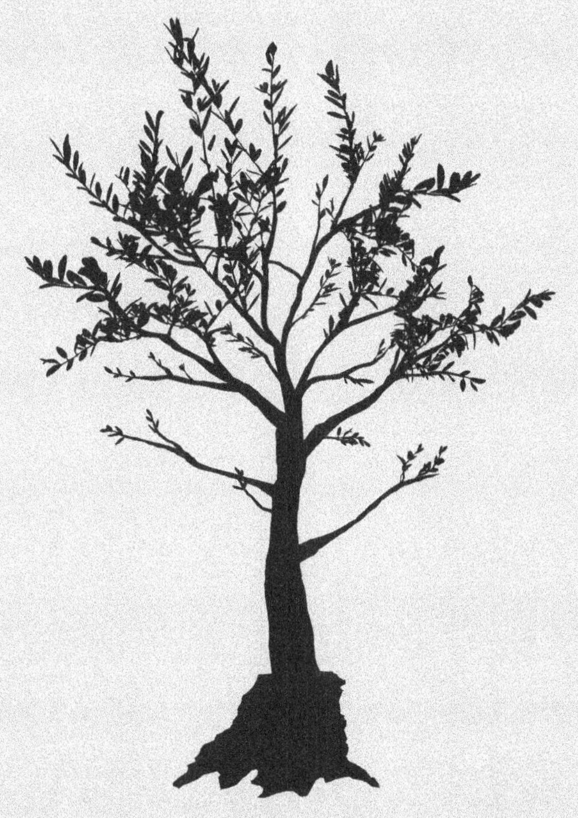

GOD SAID... *I am near.*

The Great Fish

The righteous cry out, and the LORD hears and rescues them from all their troubles. The LORD is near to the brokenhearted and saves those who are crushed in spirit. The afflictions of the righteous are many, but the LORD rescues him from them all. – Psalm 34:17–19 NASB2020

VOMITING. IT'S THE WORST! I would rather be sick with a fever or sore throat than vomit. The sensation of having your insides twist and wrench to get rid of bad food or process a virus is reminiscent of how I felt about healing. Aversion, avoidance, flight response—whatever words equate to a hard change in topic is how I was approaching my need for healing.

You may or may not be familiar with the fight-or-flight response. It's explained this way on the Psychology Tools website:

> The fight or flight response is an automatic physiological reaction to an event that is perceived as stressful or frightening. The perception of threat activates the sympathetic nervous system and triggers an acute stress response that prepares the body to fight or flee. These responses are evolutionary adaptations to increase chances of survival in threatening situations. Overly frequent, intense, or inappropriate activation of the fight or flight response is implicated in a range of clinical conditions including most anxiety disorders. A helpful part of treatment for anxiety is an improved understanding of the purpose and function of the fight or flight response.[36]

My default mode was definitely "flight" when it came to confronting healing. I may have diplomatically tried to explain my behavior as simply being pain-avoidant, but who isn't pain-avoidant? No one wants to experience pain.

When it came to writing "Part 1: The Journey," it was a challenge to relive each of those losses and feel the grief so vividly again. But I also found myself deeply encouraged by the revelation of God's persistent presence and words of hope found in His word during those times.

Writing "Part 2: The Healing" was exceedingly challenging. I didn't want to remember. Shame and humiliation were threatening to come flooding back as I remembered how bad I had allowed it to get. I rewrote this section in its entirety multiple times until I forced myself to sit in the pain again and remember what it took to come out of my darkness. In my first draft of this section, I wrote a whole lot of words offering steps or recommendations on how to go through healing. I was skirting around the vulnerable truth and not getting to the heart of it. In fact, I reread my own words and found myself getting bored and skipping over sections—not good. For the longest time, I resorted to Googling tips on anxiety and recommendations for walking through grief instead of writing my own story and experiences. I was running. I was completely terrified. That time was ugly.

It's no secret that I journal, and journaling has taught me two crucial things:

- When all my thoughts, worries, fears, concerns, life events, or experiences transfer from the whirlwind in my mind to black and white on paper, they become real and force me to take action. By "real," I mean that I have to acknowledge their existence and can no longer allow avoidance to be my default mode. Ugh.
- Writing down everything that is spinning around in my head allows me to identify which thoughts are straight-up lies from the devil. It's easier to fight a battle when the lies aren't permitted to hide in my thoughts any longer. Words on paper carry power.

It occurred to me that I was pulling a "Jonah" and running hard-core in the opposite direction of what God was calling me to do. Jonah was a minor prophet in the Old Testament who received a message of repentance and reconciliation from God for the people of Nineveh—known for committing cruelty and atrocities against Israel and other nations:

> *The word of the Lord came to Jonah... But Jonah got up to flee to Tarshish from the presence of the Lord. So he went down to Joppa, found a ship that was going to Tarshish, paid the fare, and boarded it to go with them to Tarshish away from the presence of the Lord.*
>
> –Jonah 1:1a, 3 NASB2020 (emphasis added)

> *However, the Lord hurled a great wind on the sea and there was a great storm on the sea, so that the ship was about to break up. Then the sailors became afraid and every man cried out to his god, and they hurled the cargo which was in the ship into the sea to lighten it for them. But Jonah had gone*

> *below into the stern of the ship, had lain down, and fallen sound asleep. So the captain approached him and said, "How is it that you are sleeping? Get up, call on your god! Perhaps your god will be concerned about us so that we will not perish."*
>
> –Jonah 1:4–6 NASB2020 (emphasis added)

> *So he said to them, "I am a Hebrew, and I fear the Lord God of heaven who made the sea and the dry land." Then the men became extremely afraid, and they said to him, "How could you do this?" For the men knew that he was fleeing from the presence of the Lord, because he had told them. So they said to him, "What should we do to you so that the sea will become calm for us?"—for the sea was becoming increasingly stormy. And he said to them, "Pick me up and hurl me into the sea. Then the sea will become calm for you, because I know that on account of me this great storm has come upon you." However, the men rowed desperately to return to land, but they could not, because the sea was becoming even stormier against them. Then they cried out to the Lord and said, "We earnestly pray, O Lord, do not let us perish on account of this man's life, and do not put innocent blood on us; for You, Lord, have done as You pleased." So they picked up Jonah and hurled him into the sea, and the sea stopped its raging. Then the men became extremely afraid of the Lord, and they offered a sacrifice to the Lord and made vows. And the Lord designated a great fish to swallow Jonah, and Jonah was in the stomach of the fish for three days and three nights.*
>
> –Jonah 1:9–17 NASB2020 (emphasis added)

> *While I was fainting away, I remembered the Lord, And my prayer came to You, into Your holy temple... Then the Lord commanded the fish, and it vomited Jonah up onto the dry land.*
>
> –Jonah 2:7, 10 NASB2020 (emphasis added)

Jonah knew that God would show love and compassion if Nineveh chose to repent. He refused to be the instrument God would use to bring reconciliation to the undeserving people of Nineveh. He took things into his own hands and ran as far away from God as possible. I recount the words of David in Psalm 139:7–10 (NASB2020):

> *Where can I go from Your Spirit? Or where can I flee from Your presence? If I ascend to heaven, You are there; if I make my bed in Sheol, behold, You are there. If I take up the wings of the dawn, if I dwell in the remotest part of the sea, even there Your hand will lead me, and Your right hand will take hold of me.*

There is nowhere that God isn't. Jonah had to be one stubborn dude. He chose death over obedience to God when he told the sailors to throw him overboard in the middle of a storm. He had no assurances that he would survive. Even then, God showed love and compassion on him and had him swallowed by what is described as a great fish. And then inside the belly of that great fish, Jonah sat there in the darkness and stench for three whole days before "remembering the Lord and praying." Wow.

The story of Jonah is extreme, but I was running from the thought of healing just as fiercely as Jonah ran from God. I wouldn't have described myself as running from God's presence, but in a way, I was. It took a long time to trust Him with my healing. But I found myself left with no other options. He was the only One who could reach those dark, hidden places.

The great fish that stopped me in my tracks and forced me to look up and acknowledge my need for healing turned out to be debilitating panic attacks. I couldn't function publicly anymore without a humiliating panic attack. My heart would race. I couldn't take a full breath; it felt like an elephant was sitting on my chest. I'd have to dismiss myself from meetings at work. I would sit in the car on Sunday mornings unable to get out and attend church service in person. Even being asked what I wanted for lunch or being presented with options of any kind would trigger a panic attack. Every social encounter and daily choice felt overwhelming. I couldn't function. Panic attacks were my great fish that stopped me dead in my tracks.

I couldn't run anymore. I had to fix this. I requested time away from work and took three days to tackle things head-on. I clung to God's truth in Scripture and His presence like my life depended on it—because it did. I could not get through this without Him—His love, His direction, and His healing.

Owning our story can be hard but not nearly

GO DEEPER

In this section, I reference Jonah's story and how he ran in the opposite direction after hearing a word from the Lord. Go deeper and read all four chapters in the book of Jonah. Take note of how Jonah's response to God impacted others, got him swallowed by a great fish, brought an entire nation to repentance, and resulted in a shift in focus and response to God. One additional thing to note in the story of Jonah is that even though he obeyed God, he ultimately chose to harbor bitterness and anger instead of compassion.

> as difficult as spending our lives running from it. Embracing our vulnerabilities is risky but not nearly as dangerous as giving up on love and belonging and joy—the experiences that make us the most vulnerable. Only when we are brave enough to explore the darkness will we discover the infinite power of our light.
> – Brené Brown[37]

Hopefully, you don't have to have a great fish stop you in your tracks before you take your first steps toward healing. But if you're like me and a great fish is the only way to get you to stop running, know that God is right in the middle of it.

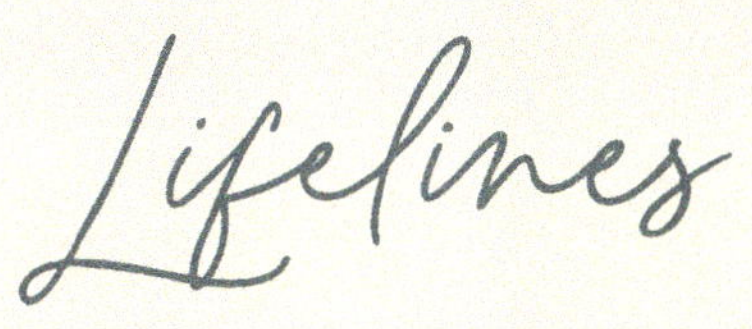

QUESTIONS TO CONSIDER

What are some reasons you might be running from healing?

Has God been trying to get your attention regarding the need for healing?

Have you encountered a "great fish" in your life? If so, what stopped you in your tracks and pointed you back to God?

SCRIPTURE VERSES

The righteous cry out, and the LORD hears and rescues them from all their troubles. The LORD is near to the brokenhearted and saves those who are crushed in spirit. The afflictions of the righteous are many, but the LORD rescues him from them all." – Psalm 34:17–19 NASB2020

Where can I go from Your Spirit? Or where can I flee from Your presence? If I ascend to heaven, You are there; if I make my bed in Sheol, behold, You are there. If I take up the wings of the dawn, if I dwell in the remotest part of the sea, even there Your hand will lead me, and Your right hand will take hold of me. – Psalm 139:7–10 NASB2020

Even though I walk through the valley of the shadow of death, I fear no evil, for You are with me; Your rod and Your staff, they comfort me. – Psalm 23:4 NASB2020

The story of Jonah in Jonah 1:1–2:10.

WORSHIP SONGS

"Breathe Life" by Jonathan Traylor from *Stones & Giants* (2018).

"I'm Listening" by Chris McClarney (featuring Hollyn) from *Music Meets Heaven*.

"Praise Before My Breakthrough" by Bryan and Katie Torwalt from *Music Meets Heaven*.

"Hills and Valleys" by Tauren Wells.

"God Will Work It Out" by Israel Houghton, Naomi Raine, and Maverick City Music.

QUOTES

"Owning our story can be hard but not nearly as difficult as spending our lives running from it. Embracing our vulnerabilities is risky but not nearly as dangerous as giving up on love and belonging and joy—the experiences that make us the most vulnerable. Only when we are brave enough to explore the darkness will we discover the infinite power of our light." - Brené Brown[38]

"The pain of recovery can often be longer and more painful than the pain of the original wounding. It's not fair but it is reality. If you are willing to partner with Jesus, you will make it through to healing and wholeness. It's hard work, but noble work and worth it." - Christine Caine[39]

BOOKS

Unashamed by Christine Caine.

PRAYER

God, thank You for Your relentless love and pursuit of me even when I was running. Your presence and Your word were the only things that sustained me. Thank You for using obstacles in my life to point me back to You—my only true source of healing and restoration. In Jesus' name, Amen.

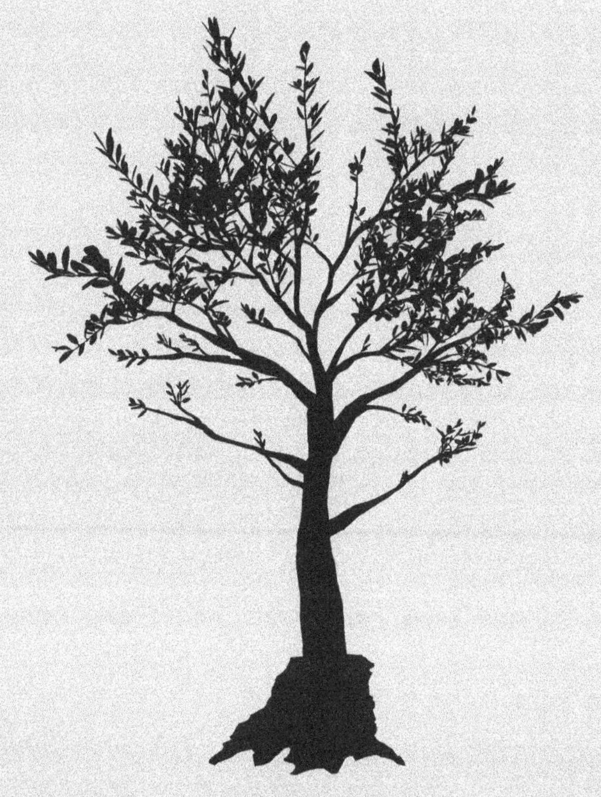

GOD SAID... *I hear you.*

Anguish Made Audible

LORD my God, I cried to You for help, and You healed me.
– Psalm 30:2 NASB2020

SOMETIMES, WHEN PAIN, ANGER, INJUSTICE, AND GRIEF STRIKE, THERE ARE NO WORDS. Your whole body shakes and vibrates from the depths of your soul, and the only thing that finds its way out is a scream! And not just any scream—we're talking about a wailing that comes from the depths. Anguish made audible.

My depths could no longer be repressed, ignored, or silenced. I had reached my capacity to overflowing. My body was revolting against me with physical symptoms—panic attacks, depression, a short fuse, binge eating, itchy welts on my hands, and an ulcer.

I wasn't sure whether I could muster the courage to open Pandora's box and confront healing head-on. The idea of healing was a topic I frequently tucked away for "later," until "later" didn't work anymore.

God reminded me about a dream He had given me a while back. In the dream, I could hear loud clanking and hammering. I was irritated that I was being disturbed by the noise. I asked God, "What is going on?" I looked up and I saw scaffolding on the moon. I asked again, "What is happening here?" He smiled and said gently, "I'm building you the moon so that your eyes won't hurt when I shed light on the dark and painful places." It was a short dream, but it showed me how well God knows me and that He knew I would need Him to walk me through the process of healing gently, step by step. Taking a bold or aggressive approach to healing would have made me withdraw even more. The assurance of this dream gave me just enough courage to take the first step and see what might happen.

GIVE YOURSELF PERMISSION TO FEEL

In the words of Elsa from Disney's Frozen, "Conceal. Don't feel. Don't let them know."[40] This became especially true for me in my experiences with grief. With every loss we experienced, I didn't feel that I had the luxury of time to fully acknowledge or face the depth of emotions bombarding my heart and soul. How do you possibly reconcile a life that has been taken from you? There never seems to be enough time to run away, scream, or mourn deeply. Life's responsibilities with family, church, work, and social obligations were always there, so what could I do?

Outwardly, I was a good friend, a smiling face, an attentive listener—the "strong" one. But on the inside, I was screaming in pain and feeling the agony of isolation and loneliness. I somehow developed this convincing facade of appearing strong. Yet if I exhaled for a moment, tears would leak down my face. Hopefully, no one noticed. Compartmentalizing the pain seemed like the most practical approach. Each time, I told myself I'd deal with it later. Time heals all wounds, right?

So many times, I preferred to wrap numbness around me like a blanket and choose to not feel. Grief felt heavy and big. It was terrifying to even consider a confrontation with grief and risk the harsh acceptance of a reality that I did not choose. While there was solace and temporary security in being numb, the unfortunate side effect was that if you choose to not feel pain, grief, or sadness, you can't feel joy, hope, or happiness either. Emotions are kind of an all or nothing deal. It's completely unfair.

I didn't see it coming, but shame jumped in with both feet as well, telling me: "You're broken. You're flawed at the genetic level. Don't cry or let your grief show. If you lose it and cry, people won't know what to do with you. You'll appear emotionally unstable. People will walk away and reject you."

Unfortunately, I ended up believing this barrage of garbage to be hard truth. I shoved my emotions down like my life depended on it. If I let the emotions from my grief leak out, it would result in ugly crying, loud sobbing, and snot everywhere; I truly believed that would result in rejection—even from those I loved the most. I didn't want to be a burden on others; they had enough going on in their own lives.

This belief shaped and defined how I managed grief. I wish I had known at the time that I was allowed to be upset and let all my emotions wash over me until they were satisfied. Sometimes, I'd find a private place to be upset, but I didn't think there was a way to share any of this with anyone else. I believed that my emotions would drive people out of my life.

I became a shell of a person. With great practice over time, I couldn't feel anything anymore. I falsely believed that numbness was preferable to falling apart every time someone showed genuine interest in how I was doing. A casual inquiry of, "How are you?" was my kryptonite. I had to figure out how to respond to the dreaded "How are you?" inquiry without feeling like I was straight up lying to people all the time. As a response, I would choose a fact like, "It was a busy week at work this week. I'm looking forward to a little extra sleep this weekend." Or I learned to pivot the conversation back to the inquirer, "Not bad. How are things going with you?" One thing was certain, it would not go well if I poured out the pain of all my failed pregnancies, social anxiety, and panic attacks to every unsuspecting inquirer. Can you even imagine?

> "Hey, how are you?"
>
> "Oh, I'm glad you asked. I'm horrible! I'm so depressed from grief and losing seven pregnancies that I struggle to feel anything anymore. I have severe panic attacks where I feel like an elephant is sitting on my chest, and I can't breathe. I'm terrified of letting any of my emotions out for fear of social rejection. I'm pretty sure I'm depressed. It took a lot to come outside today. How are you?"

This would leave any rational person bolting for the door, or maybe they'd give a polite yet awkward. "Oh, sorry to hear that." This kind of emotional vomit is not what Brené Brown was talking about when it comes to vulnerability. Even the Bible encourages us to guard our hearts.

> *Watch over your heart with all diligence, for from it flows the springs of life.*
>
> – Proverbs 4:23 NASB2020

Vulnerability starts with finding a safe place to share your heart. Even Jesus had three disciples with whom He was closer than the rest—Peter, James, and John. He shared His heart and invited them to pray with Him in His most vulnerable moments.

> *And He took with Him Peter and James and John, and began to be very distressed and troubled. And He said to them, "My soul is deeply grieved to the point of death; remain here and keep watch.*
>
> – Mark 14:33–34 NASB2020

I had isolated myself for so long that I didn't believe I had any trusted friends to confide in. I didn't know who to talk to. I couldn't handle the risk of rejection on top of what I had been dealing with. I had no idea how to get out of this darkness. I'm grateful God saw me and continued to shed light on the path out.

When my son, Jericho, was born, my heart was flooded with so much joy. He was our seventh pregnancy and the fulfillment of God's promise in Psalm 113:9:

> *He gives the barren woman a home, so that she will become a happy mother. Praise the LORD!*

God granted me my deepest heart's desire to become a mother and hold a sweet baby in my arms. Jericho opened my hurting heart and plowed through all my boundaries of self-preservation. Feeling joy again also brought out all my other emotions that I had been so careful to shove down. Although I had become a mother, I was still grieving. God was not done fulfilling His promise to me. I was on the path to learning how to be happy again.

> ### Journal Entry from March 31, 2018:
>
> I've been wondering for a while now why I feel so numb and closed off from others. I feel incapable of making close connections with others. I haven't had any close friends for years now.
>
> I was watching the television show This is Us tonight, and it occurred to me that my heart is full of grief from seven losses, which makes it very difficult to open myself up or make room for something new. I fiercely love my son and husband, but I am struggling to make room for anyone outside my family. I don't know how to let go. In a way, I am still desperately holding onto each of those precious babies we lost.

> ### Journal Entry from January 12, 2018:
>
> I'm so disappointed in myself. I had a panic attack at work today during our Friday morning meeting. I normally look forward to these meetings because it's time away from phone calls and tickets. I'm embarrassed that it happened. No one actually saw it happen. I excused myself from the meeting and went outside. The frustrating thing is that I don't know what triggered it. I feel broken. A panic attack is like noticing that I'm bleeding and not knowing where it's coming from.
>
> God, I'm afraid to ask for help or healing because I don't want to poke at where it hurts. Please give me the courage to sit through the pain so that I can live in healing. This was quite literally a moment of truth. God, what do I need to do to receive full healing from panic attacks?

Journal Entry from January 25, 2018:

I have been learning more about myself. Depression and anxiety have been creeping back. I've been wondering why my perspective has changed. I've been ashamed of my weakness and wondering why in the world my reserves are so low and why I'm not overjoyed every day knowing I have answered prayer in my arms with a living, breathing bundle of joy. This is what I have learned:

- I lost sight of who I am in Christ. My worth disappeared as I took my eyes off Jesus. My true identity got blurred, and I felt myself lose hope for my future.
- God is also trying to teach me how to feel again after all these years of shutting myself down. Learning how to feel and process emotion means feeling sad or depressed sometimes. I have a beautiful opportunity to get it right this time: embrace healing and process the emotions big or small in a healthy way—aka not shutting down and ignoring it.

Journal Entry from April 25, 2018:

God, I have been desperate for time alone with You. I miss Your presence and hearing Your voice. My heart is sad, and I can't figure out why.

Anytime that I show emotion in public, I am immediately ashamed and want to hide. I expect rejection. Emotions have never been my friend.

I'm not sure what I'm running from, but it's catching up to me. I have to come to peace with this war inside me. I'm in pain. I'm withering away on the inside. My life is starting to reflect unhealthiness. I'm overeating and gaining weight. I'm self-conscious and losing my confidence. I can push all the emotions down and distract myself with the busyness of life, but the result is not feeling anything and living in a state of numbness where my relationships stay shallow. So again, I need to do something about this torrent of emotion that is threatening to take me out. My resolve to push it all down is wavering. I deeply fear appearing crazy to others. Emotions make people look crazy sometimes. I'm just alone and at a breaking point. I need a friend in my life. I realize that I'm being fake with everyone around me while feigning happiness. But the alternative is allowing people to see how sad I am. I don't mind being vulnerable, but I don't have a solution or a way to fix this right now, so why share?

> Journal Entry from May 14, 2018:
>
> I am vulnerable with God, and I can't afford to be vulnerable with anyone else right now. I am deeply sad, and I don't have time to be sad. The annoying thing is that ignoring the sadness and choosing not to feel doesn't make it go away.
>
> God keeps whispering to my heart, "I need you to feel." He gently reminds me that He built me the moon, so that I can face the pain in soft light and not have to worry about shame. I am safe and protected. I don't have to worry about being exposed. I have no idea how to start feeling again. In my experience, emotions can't be trusted, and I especially can't trust other people with my emotions. People tell me that I need an outlet or to exercise more or to read my Bible more. Okay. I can guarantee I'm not the only one experiencing pain. What do other people do?
>
> *The LORD hears his people when they call to him for help. He rescues them from all their troubles. The LORD is close to the brokenhearted; he rescues those whose spirits are crushed. The righteous person faces many troubles, but the LORD comes to the rescue each time.*
>
> – Psalm 34:17–19

Okay, okay. I was getting the message loud and clear—embrace the emotions. Own them and find a safe place to experience all of them. Give myself permission to feel the good, the bad, and the ugly.

TV REVELATIONS

Any fans of the TV show *This Is Us*? I'm a huge fan! Every episode is raw and beautiful. I often find myself crying during the episodes. Admit it, you shed a few tears too, right? But it's okay because it's an emotional response to an amazing, well-scripted TV show that we all can relate to in some way or another. However, the truth is that *This Is Us* gives me permission to feel my own pain and let it leak out under the guise of watching TV. I experienced a huge breakthrough and revelation about my own story and healing process when watching Season 4's finale. I love how God shows up in the middle of listening to a song or watching a TV show to point and say, "This is for you. Pay attention."

Let me set up the scene. The characters Jack and Kate are celebrating the one-year birthday of the Big Three (their triplets); however, Kate is finding it difficult to celebrate because she is mourning the loss of Kyle, the third triplet, who passed away during birth. They adopted Randall, who had been dropped off at the hospital, as a brand-new infant. While they still celebrated their three babies, Kate was wrestling with the loss of Kyle. So, Jack drives them all to the hospital to see Dr. K, their OB/GYN doctor (played by Gerald McRaney) who gave them advice about turning lemons into lemonade a year ago. They hope he can share some wisdom yet again. This is how Dr. K responded to their grief:

> I think I told you last year, Jack, that my wife and I lost our first child. Well, imagine me way back then, if you can, full of hope and full of a head of hair expecting my first child. I used to sing to my wife's pregnant belly. Never had much of a voice but that didn't stop me. My go-to was Blue Skies. You know that one? "Blue skies smiling at me. Nothing but blue skies do I see. Blue bird singing a song. Nothing but blue skies from now on." And I sang that song every day to my unborn child. And then we lost that child. For the first month after that, my wife and I would sit in our den and listen to that song on our scratchy old record player over and over and over again. It made us so sad. It was like we were punishing ourselves. But then one day, my wife got pregnant again. And to my great surprise, I found myself singing that very same song to that very same belly. And then 25 years later, I danced with my daughter to that song at her wedding. That song... it made us happy; it made us sad, then made us happy again. The whole human experience just wrapped up in that one song. The hospital is kinda like that, you know. These bizarre buildings where people experience some of their greatest joys and some of the most awful tragedies—all under one roof. I think the trick is not keeping the joys and the tragedies apart. You've got to let them cozy up to one another and coexist. If you can manage to forge ahead with all that joy and heartache all mixed-up inside you, you never know which one is going to get the upper hand. But life always does have a way of shaking out to be more beautiful than tragic.
> – *This Is Us*, Season 4, Episode 18[41]

I was a weepy mess! I let those words just sink in for a few minutes. I was completely blown away. After watching this scene, my mind was playing a rapid recall of every loss and every tear cried over the last eleven years. In one raw and heartfelt speech shared by a TV doctor to a couple mourning over the loss of a baby, I finally understood that it was okay to feel joy and grief at the same time. I had always believed that you could only experience one emotion at a time. That somehow you were a crazy person if you had a slew of different emotions occurring at the same time. I'd kinda picture the Joker from *Batman*. However, that's not the case at all. As we journey through life, our experiences of heartache, joy, disappointments, and triumphs develop our emotional depth and maturity. Our life experiences allow something like a song to trigger both a smile from a happy memory and a tear remembering a heartache from the past. I felt validated and reassured. I didn't have to feel ashamed for feeling sad in remembering all the failed pregnancies when receiving a new positive pregnancy test that should bring joy. Like the doctor said on *This is Us*, I just need to let the emotions cozy up together and coexist.

Feeling multiple emotions at the same time is a badge of honor reflecting the amount of life experienced. I have experienced tragedy and loss as well as beautiful, life-changing miracles and triumphs. Shame can take a hike. Feeling this breadth of emotion at once is beautiful and well-earned.

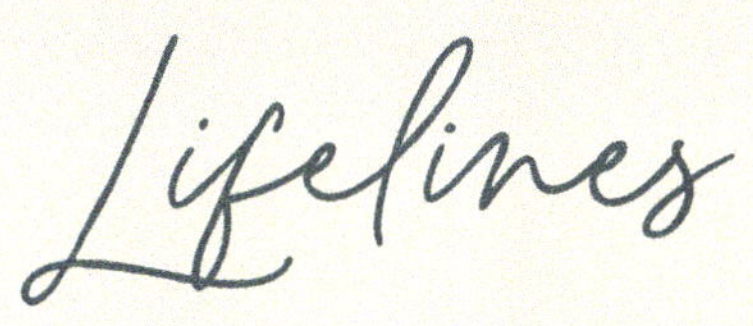

QUESTIONS TO CONSIDER

What coping methods do you resort to when it comes to grief, loss, or disappointment?

Do you trust God with your heart and your emotions? Why or why not?

Ask God to show you how to take the next step toward healing.

SCRIPTURE VERSES

The LORD hears his people when they call to him for help. He rescues them from all their troubles. The LORD is close to the brokenhearted; he rescues those whose spirits are crushed. The righteous person faces many troubles, but the LORD comes to the rescue each time. – Psalm 34:17–19

Watch over your heart with all diligence, For from it flow the springs of life.
– Proverbs 4:23 NASB2020

Bend down, O LORD, and hear my prayer; answer me, for I need your help. – Psalm 86:1

When I was in deep trouble, I searched for the Lord. All night long I prayed, with hands lifted toward heaven, but my soul was not comforted. – Psalm 77:2

I cannot keep from speaking. I must express my anguish. My bitter soul must complain. – Job 7:11 NASB2020

My eyes are swollen with weeping, and I am but a shadow of my former self... Where then is my hope? Can anyone find it? No, my hope will go down with me to the grave. We will rest together in the dust! – Job 17:7, 15–16

Trust in the LORD with all your heart; do not depend on your own understanding. Seek his will in all you do, and he will show you which path to take. – Proverbs 3:5–6

Your righteousness, O God, reaches to the highest heavens. You have done such wonderful things. Who can compare with you, O God? You have allowed me to suffer much hardship, but you will restore me to life again and lift me up from the depths of the earth. You will restore me to even greater honor and comfort me once again." – Psalm 71:19–21

WORSHIP SONGS

"Breathe Life" by Jonathan Traylor from *Stones & Giants* (2018).

"I'm Listening" by Chris McClarney (featuring Hollyn) from *Music Meets Heaven*.

"Praise Before My Breakthrough" by Bryan and Katie Torwalt from *Music Meets Heaven*.

"Hills and Valleys" by Tauren Wells.

"God Will Work It Out" by Israel Houghton, Naomi Raine, and Maverick City Music.

QUOTES

Life can get hard, and it's easy to get mired in feelings of insecurity, fear, doubt, anger and confusion. If we keep trying to preserve what only God can renew, we will continue to struggle. And then we won't be able to give anything to the lost and dying world that surrounds us. But if we go to the source Himself, if we fill ourselves daily with His living Word and refreshing presence, guess what happens? Whatever we are struggling against begins to fade away and is replaced by God's love, joy, peace and hope." - Christine Caine[42]

BOOKS

It's Not Supposed to Be This Way by Lysa Terkeurst.

PRAYER

God, thank You for being present in the middle of the healing process. Your presence and patience have gotten me through it all. Thank You for knowing me so well and protecting my heart. I can even say "Thank You" for my emotions. I'm grateful for these experiences that now allow me the privilege of comforting others. Help me to keep my eyes on You and continue to surrender as the unexpected comes my way. In Jesus' name, Amen.

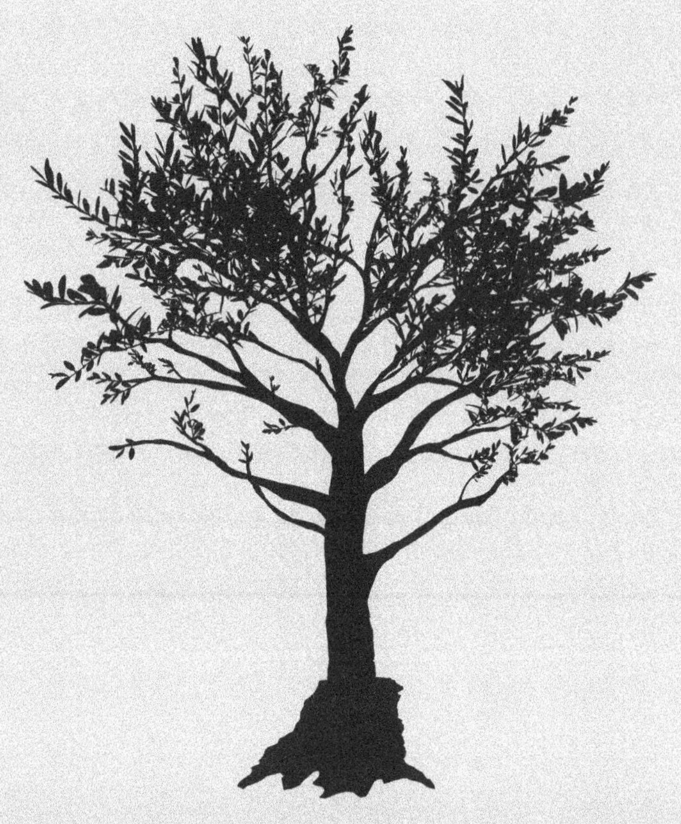

GOD SAID...

come to me. I will give you rest.

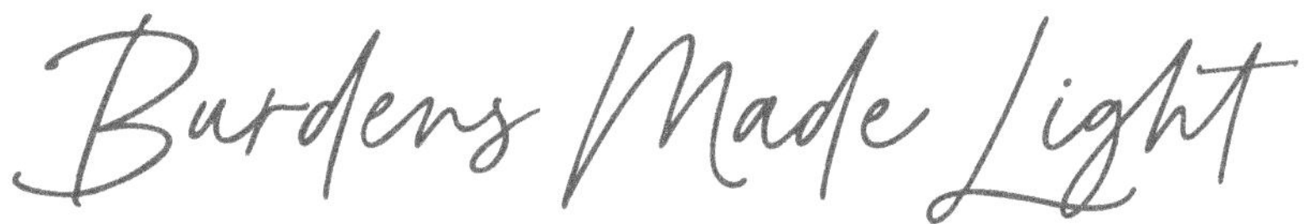

Then Jesus said, "Come to me, all of you who are weary and carry heavy burdens, and I will give you rest. Take my yoke upon you. Let me teach you, because I am humble and gentle at heart, and you will find rest for your souls." – Matthew 11:28–29

HEALING IS SUPER MESSY. It's like any big cleanup project; it gets worse before it gets better. My threshold for stuffing pain was officially broken. Panic attacks, depression, isolation, withdrawal, numbness, short fuse, crying, and more crying leaked out all over the place. What a mess! At this point, there was only one course of action left: surrender and face the mess head-on. It was time to clean up the emotional wreckage and begin the healing process. Typically, surrender has a negative connotation, which implies weakness, giving up, or losing a battle. Surprisingly, surrender carries with it a tremendous amount of freedom as well. I really missed being able to simply exhale without crying or being able to respond to the question "How are you?" without falling apart. It was time. I wanted the pain gone. I was ready to yield to what God had in mind, and I prayed the following:

God, I have to stop hiding from my pain. My heart aches so deeply. More than anything, I don't want to admit that I need healing. My whole being longs and aches to be life-giving and to nurture purpose in others. God, I know You see that. All I can say is—I surrender. Use me, God. Allow my words and actions to overflow with life from You to others. Take my pain. If I must walk through the pain, guide me step by step. Show me what I need to know, so I can share that truth with others.

> *For the Lord is the Spirit, and wherever the Spirit of the Lord is, there is freedom.*
>
> – 2 Corinthians 3:17

Surrender requires action—a relinquishing. I vowed to start with these top priorities:

- Schedule and plan a funeral for the life I expected to have.
- Trust God with my future even if it will look completely different from what I had been planning and envisioning.

STEP 1 – SCHEDULE AND PLAN A FUNERAL

I was sick with disappointment and heartache. I felt robbed. I was emotionally dragging death with me everywhere I went because I couldn't let go. There was nothing I could do to get my babies back. I decided to be intentional about giving myself a safe place to mourn and remember. I planned and scheduled a funeral and memorial service for my lost little ones.

> Journal Entry from May 14, 2018:
>
> I want to hear Your voice more clearly. I know that I have more healing ahead of me, and I appreciate Your holding my hand with every baby step bringing me closer to freedom.
>
> I listened to an amazing sermon by Christine Caine called, "The Courage to Let Go of Your Past." It was so powerful and timely! She said it plainly that healing hurts way more than the actual injury, and that we have to have the courage to make the decision to embrace the pain in its fullness in order to experience the fruit and abundant life that Jesus intended for us and wants for us. I have been in self-preservation mode. But it is becoming clear that self-preservation is preventing me from walking into the future and purpose God has for me. This is so hard!
>
> *Now glory be to God, who is able, through his mighty power at work within us, to accomplish infinitely more than we might ask or think.*
>
> – Ephesians 3:20
>
> *She is clothed with strength and dignity, and she laughs without fear of the future.*
>
> – Proverbs 31:25
>
> *You intended to harm me, but God intended it all for good. He brought me to this position so I could save the lives of many people.*
>
> – Genesis 50:20

> Journal Entry from June 12, 2018:
>
> The pain in my heart is suffocating. We're doing a memorial service for our lost babies on July 21st from 5–8 p.m. I'm terrified.
>
> - I know that I'm stuck, and I need healing in this area.
> - I'm afraid to trust others with my heartache.
> - I'm afraid to let go.
> - I feel like I might be crushed by the weight of my grief.
> - I don't like to ugly cry in front of other people.
> - I need to break my belief that emotions are a weakness.
> - I dread the thought of letting it all out and having everyone staring awkwardly in silence not knowing what to do with me.
> - I don't like being a burden or putting people out.
> - I don't like the focus being on me.
>
> *This I declare about the LORD: He alone is my refuge, my place of safety; he is my God, and I trust Him... He will cover you with his feathers. He will shelter you with his wings. His faithful promises are your armor and protection.*
>
> – Psalm 91:2, 4

I invited a few of my closest girlfriends to join me. On Saturday, July 21, 2018, we gathered in my apartment. I shared stories of my experiences with each baby. We all cried together and read Scripture verses about healing and hope. I gave myself permission to feel everything—even if it meant super ugly crying in front of my friends. I thanked God for the time I had with each one of my babies from six weeks to twelve weeks. I asked God to lavish His love on them until I could hold them in my arms someday. During this memorial service, one of my dearest friends gifted me with a pallet board painting of six olive branches. Each olive branch had a different number of leaves representing the number of weeks I was pregnant with each sweet baby. I cherish this painting more than anything! Olive branches represent new life to me—think earth after the flood. It is my hope that someday when my husband and I are able to purchase our first home, we will plant olive trees in the backyard in memory of our little ones.

Having this memorial service allowed me to breathe for the first time in years. It was exactly what I needed. I surrendered everything I was holding onto—sadness, disappointment, anger, and even the idea that having babies should be easy.

The memorial service created a lot of closure and allowed me a safe place to say goodbye. But I noticed that minor panic attacks still surfaced occasionally.

This told me that there was more surrendering to do.

STEP 2 – TRUST GOD WITH MY FUTURE

A very good friend recommended that I go to a SOZO session for healing. SOZO is basically a counseling session led by the Holy Spirit and facilitated by discerning believers who care about your healing and freedom. I was quite resistant to the idea at first. I didn't know what it would look like, and I was honestly expecting some serious ugly crying to occur. Remember that picture of the dam falling and crushing me alive? That was my expectation. I finally conceded that I should go and booked an appointment. When I arrived, I was directed to a small room in the back of the church where a couple of couches and chairs were set up. Four women were waiting in the room. The woman I had made the appointment with looked at me and said, "You have a close relationship with the Holy Spirit, don't you?" I smiled, and said, "Yes." She replied, "This is going to be easy for you." Even before we started, God was reminding me that I would not be crushed by the healing process. And that healing might not be as hard as I imagined. It might even be easy.

We simply started with prayer and allowed the Holy Spirit to guide the process. I repeated confessions of forgiveness over specific people. And it was way more than expressing forgiveness. I expressed the specific thing I was extending forgiveness for, released it back to God, and then proceeded to bless that person. I had never prayed a blessing over people who had caused me pain before. It was so freeing! And the women were taking notes of any and everything God spoke to me during that session so that I would not forget any of it later. At one point, one of them said she saw a hallway with open doors and that we needed to shut down access to Shame in my life. I told Shame it had no place in my life and to leave in Jesus' name.

I was asked to clap once and clap loud along with them on the count of three. I followed along—Three, Two, One—CLAP! In that very instant, I got a vision of a recurring nightmare I used to have. I have had vivid, horrifying nightmares my whole life—from as early as three years old and extending into adulthood. I learned how to identify the difference between a stress dream and the other ones that feel more like a personal attack or torture chamber, making the most horrific fears come to life all night long. In one of those recurring nightmares, I was being invited to a large, dark, and imposing house where friends were having a party. When I entered through the door, I could see the light of the party through a doorway over to the right and hear faint sounds of laughing and talking. But over to the left was a long dark hallway with many, many doors. And all the doors were open. I was always drawn to start walking to the left away from the party down the hallway to peer into the open doorways. At the same time, however, I was terrified to look into the doorways. I wasn't sure what I would find. It always felt like a house of shame. But at the sound of our clapping together in this SOZO session, all the doors were shut. It was incredible! Those ladies had no idea about the nightmare that I had had all those years. But Holy Spirit led them to call Shame out and remove it from my life for good. A similar experience occurred during this session in several other areas of my life. While I was expecting to be drowned in sorrow, that's not what happened at all. It was more like organizing a filing cabinet and filing misplaced grief in its proper place. Those areas of pain now had a place to go. We pulled up a "file," prayed through it, and put it where it was supposed to go and moved to the next topic. I was grateful and relieved that this part of healing looked like this for me.

I'm sure everyone's healing process will look different. It may very well come with some ugly crying, and that's encouraged. Let it all out! Emotions are healthy and God-given. I highly recommend going to a SOZO session if you're able. It made a huge difference in my healing process.

I was reminded of the man in the Bible who had been sick for thirty-eight years, which is a very long time. I can imagine that this man didn't have a lot of hope of ever being healed. And then Jesus came along.

> *Inside the city, near the Sheep Gate, was the pool of Bethesda, with five covered porches. Crowds of sick people—blind, lame, or paralyzed—lay on the porches. One of the men lying there had been sick for thirty-eight years. When Jesus saw him and knew he had been ill for a long time, he asked him, "Would you like to get well?"*
>
> *"I can't, sir," the sick man said, "for I have no one to put me into the pool when the water bubbles up. Someone else always gets there ahead of me." Jesus told him, "Stand up, pick up your mat, and walk!" Instantly, the man was healed! He rolled up his sleeping mat and began walking! But this miracle happened on the Sabbath.*
>
> –John 5:2–9

It might seem like a ridiculous thing for Jesus to ask the man if he would like to be healed, but this question makes sense to me. With any long-term trauma or condition, you come to believe that things will never change. You lose hope and stop envisioning any other reality for your life. The man tells Jesus that he doesn't have any way to get into the waters to be healed before someone else beats him to it. Too many years of trying and being disappointed. The man doesn't realize that the source of all healing is standing right in front of him. Jesus tells him to get up and walk. The man is instantly healed.

In a similar way, Jesus was asking me to get up and walk into full healing. I was nervous and not sure what life even looked like on the other side of healing. But I had nothing to lose and everything to gain. I embraced surrender again.

Journal Entry from July 6, 2022:

During my cabin retreat with God, I found myself relearning how to rest. After a four-hour nap (from nine thirty to one thirty in the afternoon), I felt a familiar panic sensation in my chest. It has always felt like a weight on my chest or like someone gripping my sternum from the inside and refusing to let go. Jesus asked me if I was ready to get rid of that, and I said, "Yes! Here take it." He replied, "I can't take grief from you. It has to be surrendered." I replied, "Then, I surrender it." But saying that wasn't enough. In my mind, I followed a chain and kept pulling and pulling and pulling until I envisioned an anchor. Grief was literally tethered or anchored to me. I wasn't totally surprised. That is exactly how it has felt. So, I asked, "Jesus, what do I do to get rid of an anchor? It is more than I can carry and too heavy to lift to get rid of on my own."

Jesus said, "I want to teach you something." I exhaled deeply and said, "Okay, I'm ready. How do we do this?"

He said, "You're looking at the wrong end of the anchor."

In my mind, I traced the anchor and followed the chain all the way back up to the source in my heart. Jesus said, "Attach the source of the anchor (the chain) to Me."

> *Then Jesus said, "Come to me, all of you who are weary and carry heavy burdens, and I will give you rest. Take my yoke upon you. Let me teach you, because I am humble and gentle, and you will find rest for your souls. For my yoke is easy to bear, and the burden I give you is light."*
>
> – Matthew 11:28–30

I wept and then laughed and said, "Well, why didn't you just say so." I have read that verse many times, but truly only heard it for the first time just now. Jesus, thank You. I don't know why You love me this much. I've been carrying this suffocating weight for so long.

Jesus said, "I need you to feel in order to share this message with others. When you are transparent with your feelings, you give others permission to feel as well."

I pictured Jesus sitting in front of me holding my left hand. Out loud, I

> told grief it no longer had a place in my life and with my right hand, I yanked at my chest as if to remove the chain and handed it to Jesus. Peace instantly fell over my body, and I felt a warm, tingling sensation in my back and shoulders.

And with that encounter, I was able to officially say goodbye to grief, panic attacks, and the hold that they had on my life. For the first time, I was able to trust God with my future and look forward to having it be completely different from what I had originally envisioned for myself.

Lifelines

QUESTIONS TO CONSIDER

If God were to ask you if you wanted to be healed, how would you respond?

Can you trust God with your future—even if it looks completely different from what you expected or planned?

Can you describe a time when you experienced the kind of rest only God can provide? If not, ask Him to show you.

SCRIPTURE VERSES

Then Jesus said, 'Come to me, all of you who are weary and carry heavy burdens, and I will give you rest. Take my yoke upon you. Let me teach you, because I am humble and gentle at heart, and you will find rest for your souls.' –Matthew 11:28–29

For the Lord is the Spirit, and wherever the Spirit of the Lord is, there is freedom." – 2 Corinthians 3:17

Now all glory be to God, who is able, through his mighty power at work within us, to accomplish infinitely more than we might ask or think. – Ephesians 3:20

"Do you want to be healed?" story. –John 5:2–9

WORSHIP SONGS

"God Will Work It Out" by Israel Houghton, Naomi Raine, and Maverick City Music.

"Breakthrough" by Chris McClarney from *Music Meets Heaven.*

"I Thank God" by Maverick City Music and UpperRoom.

BOOKS

Crushing: God Turns Pressure into Power by T. D. Jakes.

Fiercehearted by Holley Gerth.

Strong, Brave, Loved: Empowering Reminders of Who You Really Are by Holley Gerth.

PRAYER

Jesus, Your love knows no limits. You reach into the darkest of places and remind us that we do have hope and a future. Thank You for being so faithful to heal and bring restoration. We were not meant to carry such heavy burdens. I'm grateful for Your rest and that when You carry our burdens, the load is light. Surrender is the best thing I ever did. Thank You for knowing what to do with my situation, shifting my perspective, and giving me practical steps to take out of my pit. In Jesus' name, Amen.

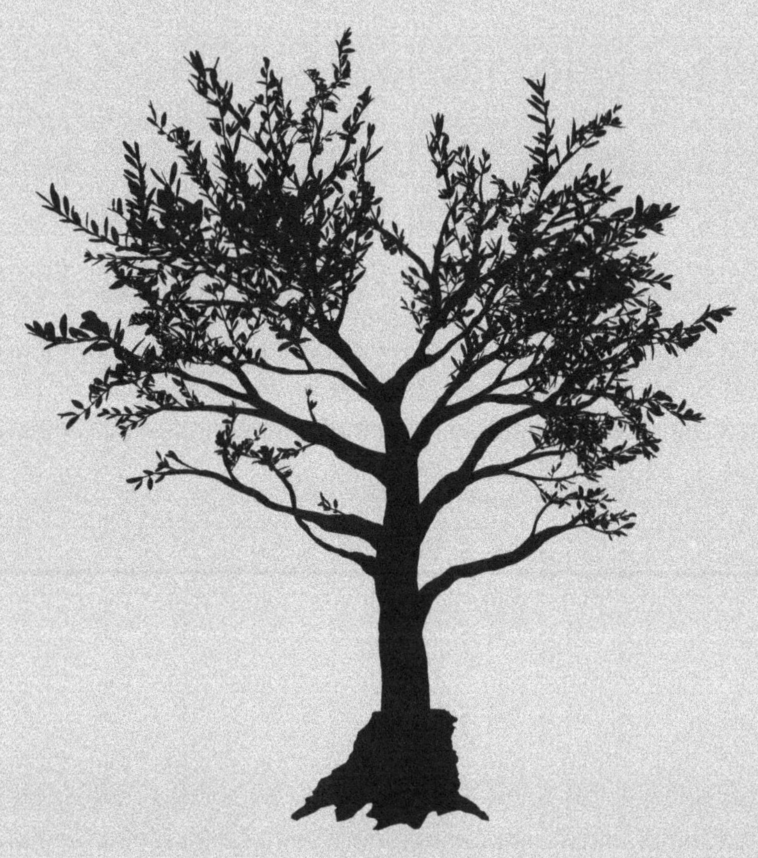

GOD SAID... *forgive.*

Freedom in Forgiveness

Get rid of all bitterness, rage, anger, harsh words, and slander, as well as all types of malicious behavior. Instead, be kind to each other, tenderhearted, forgiving one another, just as God through Christ has forgiven you.
– Ephesians 4:31–32

FORGIVENESS IS LIKE THE SWEAR WORD OF THE HEALING PROCESS. The unfortunate truth is that healing is impossible without forgiveness. The idea of "letting go" is annoying when you're in the midst of grief or deep loss. With any loss, your gut instinct is to hold tighter to everything—even anger, bitterness, or an offense.

From experience, I found the need to forgive in these three areas:

- Forgive others
- Forgive God
- Forgive myself

FORGIVE OTHERS

Many people seem to have an assumption about the appropriate threshold of time for grieving. If you surpass that threshold, people tend to express far less empathy or sympathy regarding your circumstances. In fact, responses to loss may even convey an air of "get over it" if you've been sad too long from their perspective. I try hard to put myself in their shoes. Knowing what to say to someone who is sad or grieving is challenging. You can't fix it. There probably isn't much you can do or say to make them feel better. So, what do you do?

- Send a card.
- Be present (no need to talk).

- Offer distraction with an event or a non-triggering movie.
- Drop off meals.

Well-meaning people, unfortunately, offer terrible advice. They encourage you to move on, tell you to try again, want you to stop being sad, tell you to find the positive, or change the topic altogether because they are uncomfortable with your sadness. While I understand where they are coming from and that having these encounters can be uncomfortable, it's completely unfair to put a grieving person in the position of making the other person feel better. This tends to reinforce a sense of isolation during seasons of grief.

Every empty "I'll pray for you" or "God will never give you more than you can bear" or "You're young—you can have more babies" was echoing through my mind. I would have loved to write them all off and paint myself as the victim with no obligation for surrender or restitution. I was wronged; therefore, it was their responsibility to make it right. Right? With those unfortunate experiences and memories taking up residence in my heart and mind, I was left with one annoying truth: I had to forgive. There was no way I was going to let offenses and unforgiveness keep me from freedom.

> *Search me, O God, and know my heart; test me and know my anxious thoughts. Point out anything in me that offends you, and lead me along the path of everlasting life.*
>
> – Psalm 139:23–24

The act of forgiving carries so much freedom and healing:

- Forgiveness releases the offense.
- Forgiveness removes the stress and anxiety surrounding the event.
- Forgiveness puts our focus back on God and allows us to hear His voice clearly again.

God was working on my heart. My unforgiveness was preventing healing. I asked the Holy Spirit to bring to mind every person or situation where I was holding unforgiveness. This was a brave request; it was like asking God for patience. Watch out because you'll get what you ask for! But I committed to the process and prayed:

> God, the only thing standing in the way is me. I have this laundry list of people to forgive, and I have been so stubborn. Enough is enough. I am ready for more. I pray and ask for Your help and guidance as I work through this list and release all this pain that has been holding me back.

I wrote each person's name and the situation down on a piece of paper. Let's be real. It was more like six pieces of paper. I then took the time to pray through each one and forgave them out loud one by one. Offering forgiveness out loud allows you to hear the words that you're speaking. It makes it feel more intentional and permanent. It also doesn't give the enemy any room to intervene. Praying through forgiveness included three parts:

- Confess the offense or wound out loud.
- Offer forgiveness and release the person and offense to God.
- Pray a blessing over the offender.

An example prayer of forgiveness toward others might sound like this:

> God, I felt incredibly angry, rejected, and misunderstood when Karen (fictional name) told me that I was too emotional and that I needed to stop sobbing over our losses and move on. I can't trust her or entertain the pursuit of a friendship right now, but God, I do forgive her for her callous words. I release my anger and feelings of rejection. God, You love me, and You love Karen. I ask that You bless her and somehow use this situation to show her how she can better extend Your kind of love to others in the future.

I have found that forgiveness doesn't make it feel like the incident never happened, but it does remove the sting of emotions so you can recall the incident later as a set of facts without the anger or emotional response it used to trigger.

> *Then Peter came to Him and asked, "Lord, how often should I forgive someone who sins against me? Seven times?"*
>
> – Matthew 18:21–22

My mom shared this wisdom with me on numerous occasions: "It is impossible to stay mad at people when you're praying for them." I have found this to be true. Try it and you'll see.

> *But I say to you, love your enemies and pray for those who persecute you.*
> – Matthew 5:44 (NASB2020)

> *Do not rebuke a scoffer, or he will hate you; Rebuke a wise person and he will love you.*
>
> – Proverbs 9:8 NASB2020

> *Love is patient and kind. Love is not jealous or boastful or proud or rude. Love does not demand its own way. Love is not irritable, and it keeps no record of when it has been wronged.*
> – 1 Corinthians 13:4–5 (emphasis added)

Some incidents required that I do multiple rounds of forgiveness, but I'm grateful for God's persistent nudging toward forgiveness that came through worship songs, sermons, Scripture, and my own acknowledgment and need to surrender pain in this way and let Him have it all. Carrying offenses is heavy. I could feel the weight slowly lifting.

FORGIVE GOD

Offenses left to fester lead to anger, and anger leads to bitterness. With my emotions in full force again, it was a relief to acknowledge that I was allowed to feel angry. But boy, was I angry! I had been robbed of my sweet babies. I was furious about feeling completely out of control and helpless in my own body. I was angry at the insensitivity of others, especially the church. I was angry at God.

I desperately didn't want to admit that I was angry at God. In my season of isolation and darkness, He was my only solace through each of our losses. I didn't want to risk my relationship with God by casting accusations and asking the questions that may not get answers. I found myself at an impasse. I wanted the precious babies I lost. I wanted to be the woman who didn't know loss or carry a genetic disorder. I could see that I was carrying unrealistic expectations that pregnancy should be easy or that life should magically shield me from all pain because I'm a child of God.

> God, how can You say You love me and allow me to feel so helpless and shredded on the inside? You have the power to save my babies. Do You hear me? Do You care? Why aren't You coming to my rescue? Why are You allowing so many losses to occur? Do I have to suffer this much? How bad does it have to get before You step in and help? Why don't You intervene and spare my heart? Why are You allowing this to happen to me?

My heart was screaming in anguish. David and Job had seasons in which they echoed these same questions or demanded answers from God.

> *Bend down, O LORD, and hear my prayer; answer me, for I need your help.*
>
> – Psalm 86:1

> *When I was in deep trouble, I searched for the Lord. All night long I prayed, with hands lifted toward heaven, but my soul was not comforted.*
>
> – Psalm 77:2

> *I cannot keep from speaking. I must express my anguish. My bitter soul must complain.*
>
> –Job 7:11

> *My eyes are swollen with weeping, and I am but a shadow of my former self... Where then is my hope? Can anyone find it? No, my hope will go down with me to the grave. We will rest together in the dust!*
>
> –Job 17:7, 15–16

My anger toward God and my unanswered questions were causing me to hold God at arm's length even though I didn't realize that I was doing it.

On December 5, 2015, our church had an Encounter Day to conclude our discipleship program. I was pleasantly surprised... well, that's not quite the right way to put it. I was blown away at the breakthrough that occurred. I was praying as they were inviting everyone to receive the Holy Spirit; then the pastor came over and put his hand on my forehead. The room was loud with prayer, but I heard two things: (1) "You are a warrior," and (2) "Forgive God." I've had never been told to forgive God before, so I thought I might have heard wrong. As far as being called a warrior, hearing that greatly affirmed my identity.

At the end of Encounter, they had us fill out this six-page, double-sided checklist of all the things that might be holding us in bondage. After we checked the boxes that applied to us, they invited us to receive prayer over those things and then shred the list. I ended up toward the back of the line to receive prayer. I wasn't even sure what to bring up. I had checked plenty of boxes, including depression, anxiety, anger, fear of loss, and barrenness. But I didn't have anything glaring that stood out to ask for prayer.

Holy Spirit assured me He was leading me to the right person for prayer. He was right! I ended up with Vicky. I love her to pieces. I confessed that I wasn't quite sure what to say about the list. All I knew was that I couldn't feel anything. I had shut down my emotions to the point that I couldn't have deep relationships anymore. Without having to say one more word, Vicky said, "Well yeah, you've lost multiple babies. You're grieving." And in a single moment, all the heartache that I had been holding back washed over me. The floodgates were opened. I cried loud and ugly. Vicky's hair was soaked in my tears. I felt bad, but she just held me tighter and spoke truth into my ear. She said, "Regardless of how you feel or what others say, you are a mother of beautiful babies. Even though you don't get to hold them yet, you are still a mother, and your capacity to love and mother others is great!" She also told me that I needed to forgive God.

With that being my second time hearing that, I gave pause to consider. She was right. I was angry that God's promise in Psalm 113:9 seemed to be thrown in my face with each loss. I was angry that I had to experience so many losses. I felt abandoned and left to suffer. But more than the anger I was feeling, I didn't want anything to hold me back from being able to speak life into others, and

I didn't want to let death plague my life anymore. I knew that my hope and future joy could only come from God. So, I surrendered my anger and forgave God. I vowed to trust God with His promise to me once again.

I was set free that day and walked away with a new identity of warrior and mother.

> *He gives the barren woman a home, so that she will become a happy mother. Praise the LORD!*
>
> – Psalm 113:9

> *He will cover you with his feathers. He will shelter you with his wings. His faithful promises are your armor and protection.*
>
> – Psalm 91:4

> *But my life is worth nothing to me unless I use it for finishing the work assigned me by the Lord Jesus—the work of telling others the Good News about the wonderful grace of God.*
>
> – Acts 20:24

God didn't need my forgiveness in the conventional sense because He never makes mistakes. The act of forgiving God was more about acknowledging my feelings of anger and abandonment, processing those emotions, and then releasing them. I could then allow myself to trust in His goodness and sovereignty again.

An example prayer of forgiveness toward God might sound like this:

> God, I acknowledge that You are all-knowing and all-present and that You carry all power and authority. I confess that I have been angry with You. I have felt utterly abandoned by You. It feels like You ignored my cries when I needed You most. I know that You don't make mistakes and that nothing is out of Your control, but I can't continue to carry this resentment against You. I forgive You and release it all back to You. Please take my anger. Remind me that You are present and love me. Help me to trust You with my heart and my pain. Hold my babies. Allow Your presence to wash over me. Take my past, my present, and my future. I put it all back in Your hands. Be true to Your Word and help me to believe that You do have *"plans for good and not for disaster, to give [me] a future and a hope."* (Jeremiah 29:11)

I had to let go of my need for answers and trust God with my heart and my future again. My perspective began to shift. God was showing me His hand and the power I didn't realize I had at my fingertips.

FORGIVE MYSELF

Why would I need to extend forgiveness to myself? Tragedy is outside my control, and yet there was a yearning to point the finger and hold someone or something responsible for my pain. When it came to the premature losses I experienced, I blamed myself. As a woman, I was built with the inner workings to grow, nurture, and protect a developing baby through delivery and beyond. Because of a genetic condition, I felt utterly broken and helpless to do anything about it. The finger of blame was pointed squarely in my face. My heart was crying for children of our own, and my body was betraying me. I was letting myself down. I was letting my husband down. There was no one else to blame, and shame made sure to jump in and remind me loud and clear: "You're broken."

Being diagnosed with chromosomal translocation was devastating. Our babies were losing their fight within weeks because my genetics were messed up. I was helpless to protect them. With chromosomal translocation, the chances of a successful pregnancy hinged on the luck of the draw as to which egg was fertilized. Some eggs were good, while others carried mixed-up chromosomes. We just happened to have six losses in a row before Jericho came. The fertility specialist put it coldly and simply, "You've been really unlucky." We even experienced one additional loss after Jericho.

The memorial service I described earlier helped me take a huge step closer to releasing the pain and releasing the blame I was placing on myself. The following confession of forgiveness also helped me to put things back in God's hands.

> God, I'm so ashamed. I feel so broken. I'm flawed at the genetic level. There are no hormone supplements or pills or diet adjustments that can help fix this. I blame myself for failing my unborn babies. I'm so ashamed. I know that none of this is a surprise to You. You made my innermost parts. (Psalm 139:13) So... out loud, I confess right now and choose to forgive myself for each of our losses. I break off any attachments to shame trying to tell me that I'm broken or flawed. God, You made me, and You have a plan. I release my brokenness and weakness to You because You promise that Your strength is made perfect in weakness. (2 Corinthians 12:9) I can't do anything about this genetic condition, so all that's left is to leave You room to work. Thank you for working Your glory in and out of my weakness.

Forgiveness is hard because it requires honesty. But I would rather acknowledge the truth and tackle the pain head-on than let it weigh me down and dictate my future. Anytime we surrender or release something to God, He doesn't leave a gaping hole thankfully. Instead, He is faithful to provide hope, joy, fresh perspective, rest, and the assurance that's He's got it under control.

Lifelines

QUESTIONS TO CONSIDER

Are you ready to start forgiving? Just pick one person to start. The more we can forgive, the more we release God to move and speak in our lives.

SCRIPTURE VERSES

Get rid of all bitterness, rage, anger, harsh words, and slander, as well as all types of malicious behavior. Instead, be kind to each other, tenderhearted, forgiving one another, just as God through Christ has forgiven you. – Ephesians 4:31–32

Then Peter came to him and asked, "Lord, how often should I forgive someone who sins against me? Seven times?" "No, not seven times," Jesus replied, "but seventy times seven! – Matthew 18:21–22

Search me, O God, and know my heart; test me and know my anxious thoughts. Point out anything in me that offends you, and lead me along the path of everlasting life." – Psalm 139:23–24

But I say to you, love your enemies and pray for those who persecute you.
– Matthew 5:44 NASB2020

WORSHIP SONGS

"Never Leave" by Red Rocks Worship.

"It Is Well" by Kristene DiMarco from the *You Make Me Brave (Live)* album.

"Defender" by Francesca Battistelli and Steffany Gretzinger from the *Own It* album.

"God Problems" by Maverick City Music from the *Mav Way* album.

PRAYER

Jesus, thank You for modeling what forgiveness should look like. While the act of forgiving and surrendering can be extremely challenging, I'm incredibly grateful for the freedom it brings. Help me to love myself and others in the way that You love. Give me Your eyes. Help me to see. My past, present, and future are Yours. Draw me closer and closer to You. In Jesus' name, Amen.

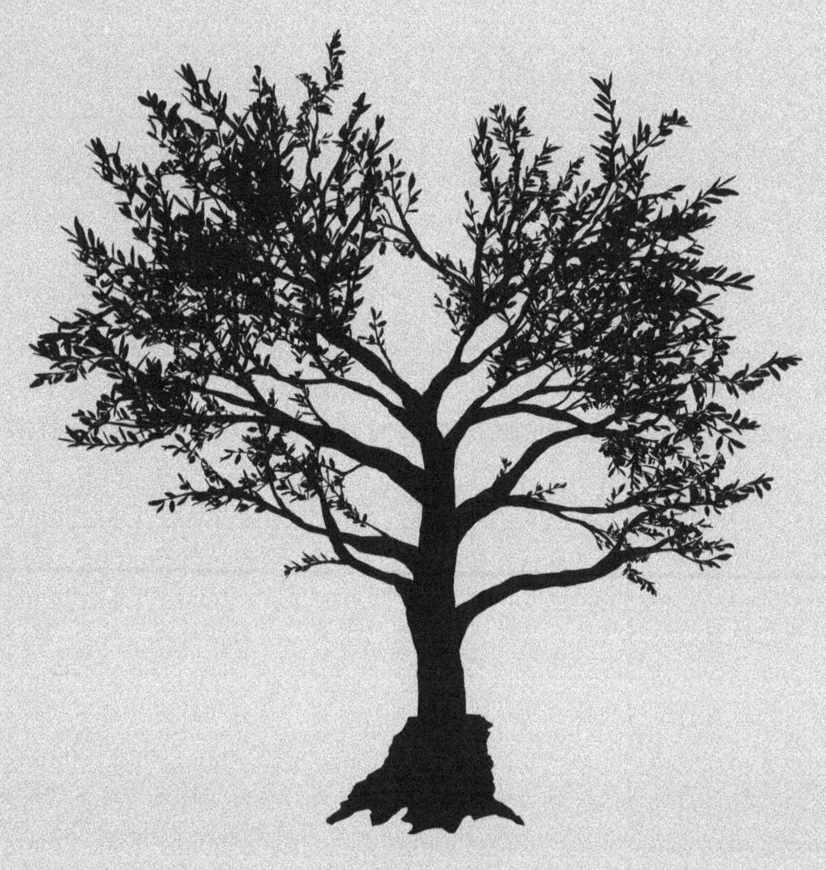

GOD SAID... *my grace is sufficient.*

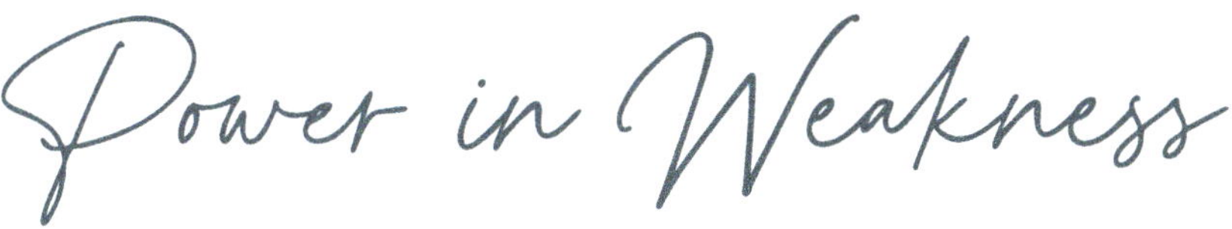

Here's the beauty of being broken: In the beginning, it always hurts. You wonder if you'll ever make it through to the other side or if any more hope lies there. The hurts and failures ride over us like waves, but once the storm has passed we see clearly again. In hindsight, we see things better than we did before. The same brokenness that shatters us, with time, brings us clarity. We stop. We reflect. We know what we need to do to move forward and make better decisions. God uses these humble and tender, broken moments to get our attention and speak to us in ways we may not have listened otherwise. – Brittney Moses[43]

IF WEAKNESS IS WHAT GOD CHOOSES TO USE, THEN HE AND I MAKE A GREAT TEAM. In college, I believed that adults should be able to take everything on themselves without needing to ask for help. I thought it was weakness or failure to need other people. But this was never God's intention. We have a Creator who continually reminds us in Scripture where our strength comes from. We were never created to do life alone.

> *But he said to me, "My grace is sufficient for you, for my power is made perfect in weakness." Therefore I will boast all the more gladly about my weaknesses, so that Christ's power may rest on me.*
>
> – 2 Corinthians 12:9 NIV

> *I pray that from his glorious, unlimited resources he will empower you with inner strength through his Spirit.*
>
> – Ephesians 3:16

> *For I can do everything through Christ, who gives me strength.*
>
> – Philippians 4:13

My struggle to be the perfect adult who didn't need anyone found immediate opposition. I found that I had a threshold of about three months before daily stresses would reach capacity. It was as if my emotions were a kettle put on the stove that slowly rose to a boil over three months until everything inside me was screaming to be removed from the heat. Once my three-month capacity was reached, I'd "lose it" for a day. "Losing it" entailed sobbing, hiding in my room, and losing the mental capacity to complete simple tasks. My mind would spin, mostly entertaining the fear of failure. It was debilitating, and I was completely mortified when this happened. In most cases, life, including school, did not wait for me. I still had papers and projects due. I didn't have the time to have a melt-down. Journaling helped, and talking with my roommate also helped. Thank God for my roommate. This pattern became a new normal for me. Life was great and manageable except for the one "freak out" day every three months or so.

Anyone who has experienced more than two minutes of adult life knows that the stresses of life become more complex, not less. My threshold of three months began to dwindle in duration over the years, and it's no surprise that my "lose it" days began to increase in frequency. Suggestions surrounding work-life balance, self-care, exercise, sleep, and diet crossed my path. All these suggestions are very good and helpful in regard to a typical, healthy routine. However, when you're feeling overwhelmed with life, the last thing you want is one more "to do" on your list. It's like saying,

> "Oh, you're feeling overwhelmed because you keep experiencing miscarriages, and you're in the middle of a busy season at work, and your husband just got laid off? Perfect! Make sure you exercise, eat right, and take time for yourself, and everything will be okay."

Work-life balance, self-care, exercise, sleep, and diet felt like new ways to fail when I was already struggling to maintain what I had on my plate. I've always been bad at asking for help. I would prefer to get stuff done myself, especially because it could be more work to try to explain what I needed to someone else. Sometimes, I didn't even know what I needed. I had to implement more of a triage process before I could even entertain the idea of integrating traditional healthy routines.

My triage process looked like this:

1. STOP and be still—even if for only five minutes.
2. Focus on breathing in and breathing out for two minutes.
3. Ask for help.
4. Talk (vent) to someone you trust or jot down everything on your mind.
5. Say "No" to anything that doesn't truly require your attention; be honest about this. Can someone else do it?

6. Determine the plan for today or even just the next hour. Tomorrow doesn't need to be figured out right now.

Along with forcing myself to stop and breathe and ask for help, I sought out safe places where I could re-center my thoughts and emotions. Journaling helped me; listening to worship music or a sermon, taking a walk, sitting in a quiet place also helped me get re-centered.

> *I love you, LORD; you are my strength. The LORD is my rock, my fortress, and my savior; my God is my rock, in whom I find protection. He is my shield, the power that saves me, and my place of safety.*
>
> – Psalm 18:1–2

When I needed this triage process, that was a red flag, a sign, that my priorities were out of balance. I was trying too hard on my own strength.

Life is surprisingly simpler when my day begins in surrender to the One who created me and knows me. I don't have to worry about failed expectations, disappointments, stresses, unexpected changes in plan, or bad news. The reason I don't have to worry is because I give it all to God before my day even starts. I say out loud, "God, I need You. I trust You. This day and everything in it are Yours. Use me. Allow me to be a light to others. I'm Yours." This prayerful surrender of the day to God in the morning sets me up for success. My identity as a child of God is reaffirmed, and I feel untouchable. My mind is at peace, regardless of the stresses the day may bring. The act of acknowledging that God is in control allows me the freedom to experience out-of-control events without the weight of the worry and stress. God has my back, my sides, and my front.

Psalm 139:1–18 summarizes it perfectly:

> *O LORD, you have examined my heart and know everything about me. You know when I sit down or stand up. You know my thoughts even when I'm far away. You see me when I travel and when I rest at home. You know everything I do. You know what I am going to say even before I say it, LORD. You go before me and follow me. You place your hand of blessing on my head. Such knowledge is too wonderful for me, too great for me to understand! I can never escape from your Spirit! I can never get away from your presence! If I go up to heaven, you are there; if I go down to the grave, you are there. If I ride the wings of the morning, if I dwell by the farthest oceans, even there your hand will guide me, and your strength will support me. I could ask the darkness to hide me and the light around me to become night—but even in darkness I cannot hide from you. To you the night shines as bright as day. Darkness and light are the same to you. You made all the delicate, inner parts of my body and knit me together in my mother's womb.*

> *Thank you for making me so wonderfully complex! Your workmanship is marvelous—how well I know it. You watched me as I was being formed in utter seclusion, as I was woven together in the dark of the womb. You saw me before I was born. Every day of my life was recorded in your book. Every moment was laid out before a single day had passed. How precious are your thoughts about me, O God. They cannot be numbered! I can't even count them; they outnumber the grains of sand! And when I wake up, you are still with me!*

And the best part is that nothing can separate me from God. He is in control when everything feels out of control.

No, despite all these things, overwhelming victory is ours through Christ, who loved us. And I am convinced that nothing can ever separate us from God's love. Neither death nor life, neither angels nor demons, neither our fears for today nor our worries about tomorrow—not even the powers of hell can separate us from God's love. No power in the sky above or in the earth below—indeed, nothing in all creation will ever be able to separate us from the love of God that is revealed in Christ Jesus our Lord.

– Romans 8:37–39

MARY AND MARTHA

> *Now as they were traveling along, He [Jesus] entered a village; and a woman named Martha welcomed Him into her home. And she had a sister called Mary, who was also seated at the Lord's feet, and was listening to His word. But Martha was distracted with all her preparations; and she came up to Him and said, "Lord, do You not care that my sister has left me to do the serving by myself? Then tell her to help me." But the Lord answered and said to her, "Martha, Martha, you are worried and distracted by many things; but only one thing is necessary; for Mary has chosen the good part, which shall not be taken away from her."*

– Luke 10:38–41 NASB2020

Martha invites Jesus into her home, but she gets swept up in the duties of hospitality. Exasperated at her sister, Martha vents to Jesus asking Him to make her sister help with serving their guests. It's very sweet that Jesus calls her by name twice to get her full attention and assures her that He hears what she is saying. He acknowledges that there is a lot on her plate, but then shifts her perspective and reminds her that her sister, Mary, has chosen what is better—soaking in every word from the Lord.

Growing up in the church, this story always felt like a woeful tale of caution: "Don't be like Martha. Be more like Mary." Mary's choice to sit at Jesus' feet and soak in His words is absolutely a good thing. But then I'm left wondering, what would have happened to all the preparations had Martha done the same thing? No one would have had food to eat or drink. What is Jesus trying to say here? Shirk all your responsibilities and sit in His presence all the time? I suspect not. Jesus pointed out that Martha was "worried and distracted about many things." Reading that phrase again suddenly made this passage very personal. I am 100 percent guilty of allowing my mind to spin and spin on "many things." And these "things" keep my focus off Jesus. He was right to correct her and remind her where her focus should be. Jesus was helping Martha learn how to shift her focus and trust Him when life feels too heavy and overwhelming. Power in weakness 101 straight from Jesus.

Lifelines

QUESTIONS TO CONSIDER

How do you feel about weakness?

Describe a time when God's power was shown through your weakness. If you haven't yet experienced His power in your weakness, invite Him into your weakness now and see what He can do.

SCRIPTURE VERSES

I love you, Lord; you are my strength. The Lord is my rock, my fortress, and my savior; my God is my rock, in whom I find protection. He is my shield, the power that saves me, and my place of safety. – Psalm 18:1–2

But he said to me, 'My grace is sufficient for you, for my power is made perfect in weakness.' Therefore I will boast all the more gladly about my weaknesses, so that Christ's power may rest on me. – 2 Corinthians 12:9

I pray that from his glorious, unlimited resources he will empower you with inner strength through his Spirit. – Ephesians 3:16

For I can do everything through Christ, who gives me strength.
– Philippians 4:13

WORSHIP SONGS

"You Are My Champion" by Dante Bowe from the *Champion (Live)* album.

"In the Name of Jesus" by JWLKRS Worship and Maverick City Music.

SERMONS

"The Courage to Let Go of Your Past" by Christine Caine. YouTube Link: https://www.youtube.com/watch?v=NkNLGASZM7k&t=4s.

BLOG

"A Journey of Faith & Mental Wellness – 5 Qualities of the Authentically Strong" (blog) by Brittany Moses, https://brittneyamoses.com/5-qualities-authentically-strong.

PRAYER

Jesus, thank You that Your grace is sufficient. I'm sorry for my stubbornness in trying to carry all the weight of life on my own. I'm sorry for not asking for help or surrendering my load to You sooner. Thank You for being able to use my weakness to display Your strength. I'm grateful that Your presence is all that I need. In Jesus' name, Amen.

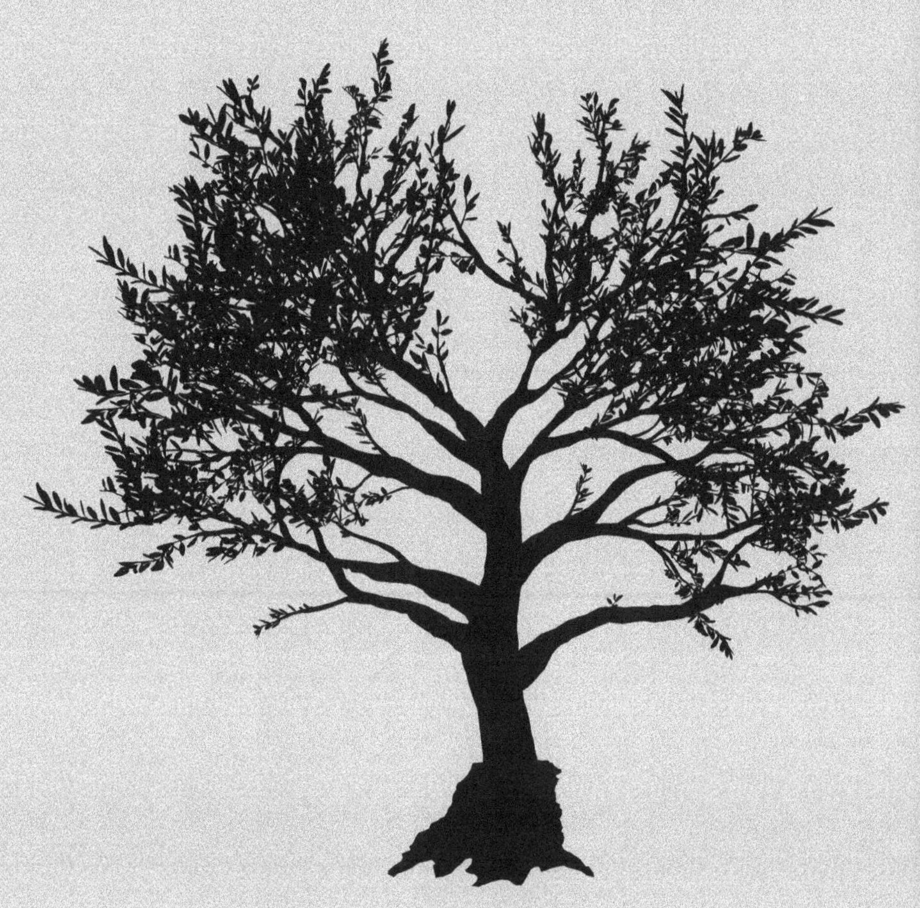

GOD SAID... *encourage one another.*

Strength in Numbers

Let's hold firmly to the confession of our hope without wavering, for He who promised is faithful; and let's consider how to encourage one another in love and good deeds, not abandoning our own meeting together, as is the habit of some people, but encouraging one another; and all the more as you see the day drawing near. – Hebrews 10:23–25 NASB2020

PEOPLE WHO WORK IN CUSTOMER SERVICE joke that customer service would be a breeze if it weren't for the customers. If you've ever worked a day in customer service, you get it. A good friend of mine described it perfectly: people are messy. And she's right. People are messy. We strive to make good impressions and paint a facade that we somehow have it all together all the time. Social media is evidence of this. The truth is that maintaining the facade is exhausting, and most of us crave genuineness and connection. But there is great risk in being vulnerable; people might see our mess and then what? Fear of rejection is a powerful deterrent to vulnerability. However, without vulnerability, true connection cannot happen. The alternative is isolation. I'm grateful for all the research Brené Brown has done on the concepts of vulnerability and connection.

> I define connection as the energy that exists between people when they feel seen, heard, and valued; when they can give and receive without judgment; and when they derive sustenance and strength from the relationship.
> – Brené Brown[44]

I readily admit that I struggle to be vulnerable because I so desperately want to hide my mess. The approval of others and avoiding rejection are strong forces in my life. Additionally, the layers of unresolved grief that I carried, without any means to express or release it, further contributed to my reluctance to share my struggles.

Over the span of eleven years, I experienced the pain of seven miscarriages (six before Jericho and one after), and this accumulated into emotional baggage comparable to that of a hoarder, making it nearly impossible to navigate socially without stumbling or knocking over piles of emotional weight.

I found myself in an unhealthy pattern making concessions to pain instead of confronting it head-on. I couldn't let anyone see me this way. I was humiliated, but I was also too tired to tackle this mountain alone.

Grief is isolating and makes you want to hide. It draws you inward. And it's in that space that I found myself taking residence. I wanted to ask for help, but fear of rejection kept me silent and alone. Remaining inwardly focused, wrapped up in my own thoughts, fears, and worries led to social paralysis. I recognized that this inward spiral distanced me from others and a deeper connection with God, leaving me on the brink of losing hope.

On evenings when I found myself alone with my thoughts, I felt the weight of it all. I wanted to cry, scream, or call someone to come and help me. But I didn't know who to call or text. People are busy, and I didn't want to trouble them with my problems. I would tell myself to rely on God as my refuge, my ever-present help in trouble, and my rock. I was tempted to feel shame for wanting someone to sit with me instead of doing the more "spiritual thing," spending more time in prayer. But God hard-wired us for community. There is no shame in needing each other; healing comes when we share our burdens out loud. It helps us to process the situation when we confess our pain and accept its reality. We also realize that we are not alone. Thank goodness!

> *Share each other's burdens, and in this way obey the law of Christ.*
>
> – Galatians 6:2

> *Two people are better off than one, for they can help each other succeed.*
>
> – Ecclesiastes 4:9

> *Confess your sins to each other and pray for each other so that you may be healed. The earnest prayer of a righteous person has great power and produces wonderful results.*
>
> –James 5:16

> *So it is with Christ's body. We are many parts of one body, and we all belong to each other.*
>
> – Romans 12:5

> *For where two or three gather together as my followers, I am there among them.*
>
> – Matthew 18:20

Blessed be the God and Father of our Lord Jesus Christ, the Father of mercies and God of all comfort, who comforts us in all our affliction so that we will be able to comfort those who are in any affliction with the comfort with which we ourselves are comforted by God.

– 2 Corinthians 1:3–5 NASB2020

Therefore encourage one another and build up one another, just as you also are doing.

– 1 Thessalonians 5:11

Why was I terrified of the thing I needed most? I knew it was important for me to go back to church. We need community. God designed us for fellowship and relationship. Community allows for shared experiences, laughter, comfort, support, friendship, and love. But it also opens us up to rejection, hurtful words and opinions, and ironically, an acute sense of isolation when we don't fit in. Although I wanted to find a way to open myself to others and embrace community in hopes I could trust a few good people, I also wanted to remain guarded just in case. Unfortunately, you can't be both trusting and guarded. How was I going to move forward? Was I ready for community? No idea. But I had to find out.

Surrender and vulnerability were the keys for me to find the courage to step back into community. At the heart of genuine connection lies vulnerability—a willingness to open oneself up. Yet, vulnerability is not easily granted, as trust must be earned. As we established earlier, people are messy, and that makes trust a scarce and precious commodity. However, my heart was yearning for connection.

Then the LORD God said, "It is not good for the man to be alone; I will make him a helper suitable for him."

– Genesis 2:18 NASB2020

Rejoice with those who rejoice, and weep with those who weep.

– Romans 12:15 NASB2020

Do nothing from selfishness or empty conceit, but with humility consider one another as more important than yourselves; do not merely look out for your own personal interests, but also for the interests of others.

– Philippians 2:3–4 NASB2020

"With all humility and gentleness, with patience, bearing with one another in love."

– Ephesians 4:2 NASB2020

And if one can overpower him who is alone, two can resist him. A cord of three strands is not quickly torn apart.

– Ecclesiastes 4:12 NASB2020

We urge you, brothers and sisters, admonish the unruly, encourage the fainthearted, help the weak, be patient with everyone.

– 1 Thessalonians 5:14 NASB2020

I watched a sermon by Pastor Steven Furtick at Elevation Church illustrating the power of community. It was about the widow's olive oil in 2 Kings 4. The widow came to Elisha the prophet begging and pleading for help. Her deceased husband's debtors were coming to collect her two sons as slaves. I can't even imagine! Talk about going through a season of being kicked while you're down. Her husband dies, she's stuck with all his debt, and now she's about to lose both her sons as slaves to debtors. Elisha instructed her to go to her neighbors to collect as many jars as she could and then go into her home, shut the door, and pour her little olive oil into the jars she had collected. All the jars ended up full. You read that correctly. God used the little olive oil she had and enlarged her provision. As she was filling the last jar, the flow of the oil stopped, and she was instructed to sell the jars of oil to pay the debts.

God can use the little we have if we trust Him with it, but more than that I love how this story highlights the importance of community. The widow reached out to her neighbors to collect as many jars as possible. We might think we're alone, but we only need to muster the courage to ask for help and trust God with the rest.

A LOSS AND A BREAKTHROUGH

Five months after Jericho was born, we were surprised with a positive pregnancy test. I had my suspicions that I might be pregnant again with the symptoms I was experiencing. We scheduled a doctor appointment and started the waiting game, hoping and praying everything would be okay. We didn't quite make it. We lost our sweet baby #7 at six weeks old.

Everything I had learned after so many previous losses seemed to get thrown out the window. You'd think I would know how to process and heal in a healthy way by now, but I was struggling. I wanted to declare hope and remind myself of God's faithfulness, but I felt numb and defeated. I forced a smile on my face and walked through the motions of life again, but my heart was weeping. Panic attacks returned and attending church and being around people felt overwhelming to me—again! My insides ached with this all too familiar weight of grief.

During this time, my community surprised me. My work family showed so much love and support. They sent us flowers and left dinner at our doorstep. They also told me to take a few days off and rest. I was overwhelmed with gratitude at the generosity.

I had to take it one day at a time. I let the words of worship songs wash truth over my heart and soul. I leaned in to hear the voice of God and clung to Him for comfort.

I sincerely wrestled with forcing myself to connect with other believers again after a long season of grieving in silence. I struggled with the inevitable question, "How are you doing?" This dreaded question was my social kryptonite. I never knew how to respond. Should I say, "I'm doing great. Wonderful!" and hope they didn't catch the insincerity in my eyes? Did they really want to know how I was doing, or was it a social courtesy to ask? I wasn't sure. But even with all the uncertainty, I faced my fears and attended church. I made it through the doors with minimal interactions—thank, goodness! I found a seat and eagerly waited for service to begin. And then an amazing thing happened. Service started with a Bethel song called "King of my Heart." Our church almost never sang songs from other churches. The most beautiful thing about that song was that God brought it to my attention via YouTube Music five days earlier. I'd been playing it nonstop the entire week. Hearing that song at church was the biggest hug from God I could've received. It was an assurance that He saw me. I even had someone come and put her arms around me and pray that I would be filled with hope and joy. She prayed against loneliness and depression and anxiety. She spoke life into me and over me. I walked away feeling exhausted and deeply encouraged. I survived my first encounter with community, and it was a success.

> *This I declare about the LORD: He alone is my refuge, my place of safety; he is my God, and I trust him.*
>
> – Psalm 91:2

As an introvert going through healing, connection was incredibly difficult. I was still convinced that if I was vulnerable and shared my pain with someone else, that it would result in rejection. I didn't feel like my emotions could be trusted at all. I asked God to bring safe people into my life. I practiced social interactions again on Sunday mornings at church. Despite all my inner protests and apprehension, we ended up hosting a small group Bible study at our apartment. It seemed like a good first step to invite folks to our place. These encounters slowly taught me that there are people who can be trusted. Repeated exposure in these safe environments helped me to build the courage to ask for help or prayer when I needed it. The amazing thing is that I never once encountered rejection for my acts of vulnerability. It took practice and time, but I began to see how doing life with others was completely God's design. My inward focus shifted, and I found the courage to lift my head. The community I encountered helped me to look outward and upward. I listened to others tell their stories of God's faithfulness in hard times, and my hope was reborn. For the first time in years, I didn't feel stuck in my isolation. I could see a way forward, focused on Him and surrounded by friends who kept pointing me back to Him.

The church community is a true blessing and extension of family. These meaningful friendships and godly connections are essential, because when life blinds you from the One, you have people in your corner who can remind you of God's faithfulness, especially during your darkest moments. We all need people who aren't afraid to confront us when needed and urge us to let go of negativity, immerse ourselves in worship music, and recall the magnitude of the God we serve. Church family helps us to redirect our focus from ourselves back onto Him. Our spirits are encouraged, and our perspective is renewed. When believers come together, watch out! You suddenly have people united under God fighting on your behalf.

Lifelines

QUESTIONS TO CONSIDER

How has community impacted your healing journey?

Do you have safe believers in your life that you can trust with the hard things? If not, ask God to bring safe people into your life—people who can help support you on your healing journey. We need each other.

SCRIPTURE VERSES

Two are better than one because they have a good return for their labor. For if either of them falls, the one will lift up his companion. But woe to the one who falls when there is not another to lift him up." – Ecclesiastes 4:9–10 NASB2020

Blessed be the God and Father of our Lord Jesus Christ, the Father of mercies and God of all comfort, who comforts us in all our affliction so that we will be able to comfort those who are in any affliction with the comfort with which we ourselves are comforted by God. – 2 Corinthians 1:3–5 NASB2020

So it is with Christ's body. We are many parts of one body, and we all belong to each other. – Romans 12:5

For where two or three gather together as my followers, I am there among them. – Matthew 18:20

And let us not neglect our meeting together, as some people do, but encourage one another, especially now that the day of his return is drawing near.
– Hebrews 10:25

SERMONS

"Frozen Oil and Chosen Vessels" by Steven Furtick, Elevation Church, https://elevationchurch.org/sermons/frozen-oil-and-chosen-vessels.

BOOKS

Unburdened: Stop Living for Jesus So Jesus Can Live Through You by Vance Pitman. It highlights the importance of community and why God created us to do life together.

PRAYER

God, please bring safe Jesus followers into our lives. Allow us to share our burdens with one another and encourage each other. Remind us that we are never alone. Please show us the value of doing life together and help us to be brave in asking for help when we need it. Thank You for designing us to be relational. Thank You in advance for bringing meaningful and genuine relationships into our lives. In Jesus' name, Amen.

Healing in Hindsight

As I said at the beginning of this section, the blessings I experienced coming out of my darkness caught me by surprise. I had lost so much, but God was faithful to restore above and beyond anything I could have imagined. I learned that I wasn't powerless.

Practically speaking, my journey through healing encompassed:

- Running from the very healing I needed.
- Confronting the anguish that was burdening my heart and soul.
- Embracing the depths of my emotions.
- Letting go and trusting God with an unknown future.
- Extending copious amounts of forgiveness.
- Discovering the importance of self-care.
- Reconnecting with and embracing the support of a loving church community.

Looking back, if I could boil my healing journey down to one thing that made ALL the difference in the world, what would it be? What allowed me to continue to hope? What empowered me to look up instead of drown in sorrow? I can honestly point to one thing - JESUS. Ultimately, my hope, strength, and restoration came from being rooted in the presence of Jesus. While coping mechanisms may have offered temporary reprieve, they always fell flat in comparison to the love, healing, and comfort I found in Jesus. He alone was able to take my brokenness and transform it into something new and beautiful.

> *For I am about to do something new. See, I have already begun! Do you not see it? I will make a pathway through the wilderness. I will create rivers in the dry wasteland.*
>
> – Isaiah 43:19

One word and even one whisper from Jesus speaks life, truth, identity, and wholeness. I am grateful beyond words for His goodness and faithfulness. I am humbled that He saw me and continues to see me. He truly holds my heart, my dreams, my passions, my past, my present, and my future, and I freely give them to Him. Healing may be instantaneous for some or a process over many years for others, but it does not have to be complicated. Healing is simple: Sit in His presence. That's it. His presence is what will transform your life. Jesus is our advocate, defender, friend, and the lover of our souls.

> *I will be glad and rejoice in your unfailing love, for you have seen my troubles, and you care about the anguish of my soul. You have not handed me over to my enemies but have set me in a safe place.*
>
> – Psalm 31:7–8

part 3 | The Revelation

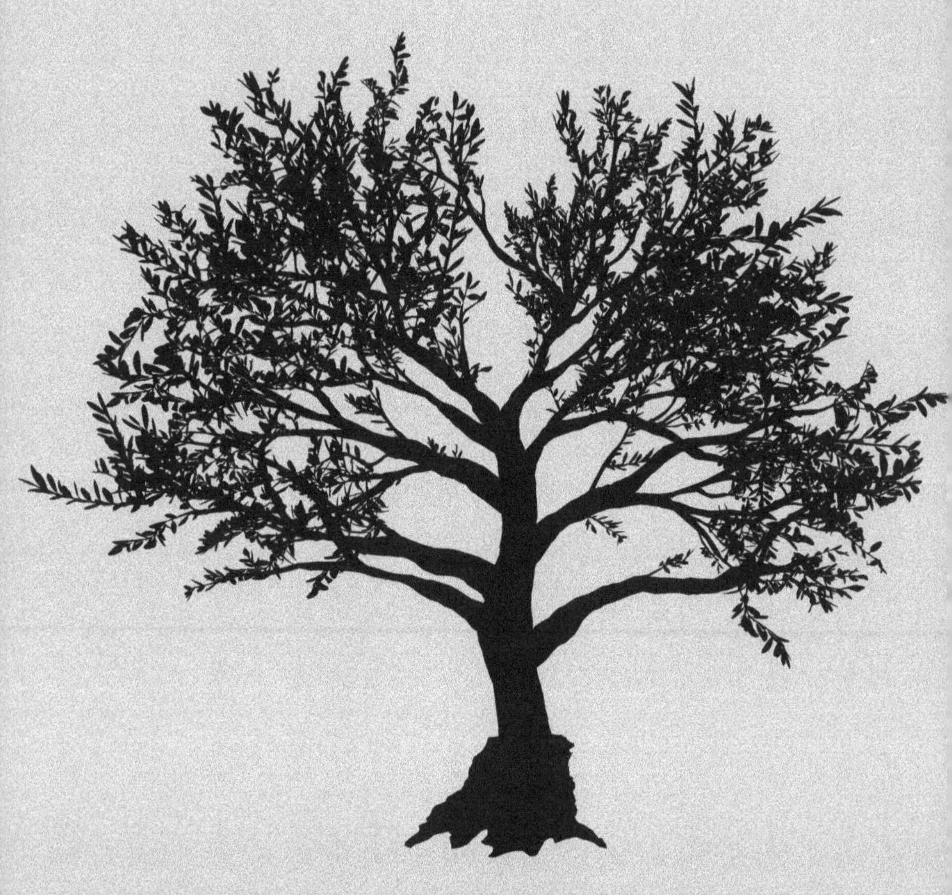

GOD SAID...

be strong in the strength of My might.

Stand Firm

Finally, be strong in the Lord and in the strength of His might. Put on the full armor of God, so that you will be able to stand firm against the schemes of the devil. For our struggle is not against flesh and blood, but against the rulers, against the powers, against the world forces of this darkness, against the spiritual forces of wickedness in the heavenly places.
– Ephesians 6:10–12 NASB2020

YOU CAN RECEIVE EMOTIONAL HEALING, KICK SHAME TO THE CURB, FORGIVE, AND EMBRACE COMMUNITY, but still experience triggers that tempt you to walk back into old habits of grief and isolation. The only way to overcome this tendency is to equip yourself with the tools and weapons you need to stand firm, fight back, and declare freedom.

In the very beginning of this book, I said: Words are powerful. Words spoken by God part the seas, bring the dead back to life, heal the blind and crippled, multiply provisions (fish and loaves), and cause the barren woman to bear children. Hold onto the words of God.

> *For the word of God is living and active, and sharper than any two-edged sword, even penetrating as far as the division of soul and spirit, of both joints and marrow, and able to judge the thoughts and intentions of the heart.*
>
> – Hebrews 4:12 NASB2020

> *And you will know the truth, and the truth will set you free.*
>
> –John 8:32 NASB2020

Life will inevitably throw stressors our way and tempt us to pick up our old self-sabotaging habits of coping—binge eating, compulsive spending, excessive sleeping, excess alcohol or caffeine, or the tendency to avoid the issue altogether. The Bible confirms that we will have tribulation in this life, but we are also reminded that God is our source of help. When we are rooted in Him and His truth, we have peace in the midst of any storm or obstacle that comes our way. Healing takes courage. No matter what comes your way, remember your source. Victory is already yours.

> *These things I have spoken to you so that in Me you may have peace. In the world you have tribulation, but take courage; I have overcome the world.*
>
> –John 16:33 NASB2020

We are not powerless or defenseless. We have been equipped with tools to fight depression, grief, and so much more. Know your enemy. Gain wisdom. Stand firm. Fight.

Grief had me believing that I was stuck and that there was no hope; the grief felt too big to tackle and overcome. I wasn't sure how to crawl out of the darkness. But my Savior did exactly what He said He would in my dream; he shed light on my next step and then the next step and the next one after that. But reading through my old journal entries showed me something truly magnificent! I found a pattern. In every moment of loss, I inadvertently resorted to the weapons in my arsenal. I didn't even realize I was doing it. It used to drive me crazy when people would commend me for being so strong because I didn't feel strong. I was only doing what I knew to survive and for me, that meant grasping and clinging to God.

Although I suffered debilitating heartbreak, I discovered that I was never powerless—ever! I don't have a five-step magic recipe to help remove your pain of grief and loss, but I can point you to the strength and hope I found. You are not powerless! I learned to fight back with three powerful weapons: prayer, the word of God, and worship.

PRAYER

> *Don't worry about anything; instead, pray about everything. Tell God what you need, and thank him for all he has done. Then you will experience God's peace, which exceeds anything we can understand. His peace will guard your hearts and minds as you live in Christ Jesus.*
>
> – Philippians 4:6–7

Prayer may seem intimidating depending on how you grew up and how you were introduced to it. Maybe it's completely foreign to you. Thankfully, prayer is simple; it is simply a conversation with God. It is an exchange of talking and listening. It's a relationship. There isn't a formula or magic combination of words that makes one prayer better than another. Prayer is telling God how awesome He is. It's asking God to join you in whatever you're experiencing. It's telling Him about your day and the things that excite you or the things that weigh you down. It's pressing in and listening to His voice, an impression, an answer, a Scripture verse, a song on the radio, or an encouraging word from a friend. God's words carry power, and they change everything.

If the concept of having a conversation with God is new to you, remember that all conversations and relationships begin with an introduction. Let me introduce you.

WHO IS GOD?

God created the heavens and earth. He created light, darkness, the sun, the moon, stars, galaxies, planets, land, bodies of water, animals, birds, fish, people—everything. If we stop long enough to experience His creation, we will realize that everything around us speaks of God's greatness. The purpose of God's original design was to have relationship with His creation, but we separated ourselves from God by sin (any act against the nature of God). Light and darkness cannot share the same space. In the same way, the holiness of God cannot share space with sin. Our sin broke God's heart, but His love for us would not allow us to remain separated from Him forever. He made a way back to Himself through Jesus.

> *For God so loved the world that he gave his one and only Son, that whoever believes in him shall not perish but have eternal life. For God did not send his Son into the world to condemn the world, but to save the world through him.*
>
> –John 3:16–17 NIV

God's heart is for salvation, not condemnation. When you accept Jesus into your life, your connection with God is restored. You become righteous, holy, forgiven, and in right standing with God. To get a glimpse at the scope of who God is, take a look at some of the ways God is described in the Bible:

- Alpha and Omega (Revelation 1:8)
- Banner (Song of Solomon 2:4)
- Creator (Genesis 1:1, John 1:3)
- Faithful (Deuteronomy 7:9, Lamentations 3:23)
- Father (Psalm 68:5)
- Friend (John 15:15)
- Healer (Psalm 103:2–5)

- Holy (Isaiah 6:3)
- Light (1 John 1:5)
- Lord (Deuteronomy 6:4, Psalm 146:5)
- Love (1 John 4:7–21) Omnipresent (Jeremiah 23:24)
- Omnipotent (Isaiah 40:28)
- Omniscient (Psalm 139:1–3)
- Provider (Philippians 4:19)
- Redeemer (Zephaniah 3:17, Psalm 18:1–2)
- Savior (Romans 10:9)
- Shepherd (Psalm 23:1, John 10:27)

WHO IS MY ENEMY?

When God created the world, He also created angels. Angels are spiritual beings that the Bible describes as warriors, guardians, and messengers. They have specific roles and characteristics with one thing in common—to worship God and minister to His people. Among the angels was Lucifer—a mighty angelic guardian of light. This is how he is described:

> *You were the model of perfection, full of wisdom and exquisite in beauty. You were in Eden, the garden of God. Your clothing was adorned with every precious stone—red carnelian, pale-green peridot, white moonstone, blue-green beryl, onyx, green jasper, blue lapis lazuli, turquoise, and emerald—all beautifully crafted for you and set in the finest gold. They were given to you on the day you were created. I ordained and anointed you as the mighty angelic guardian. You had access to the holy mountain of God and walked among the stones of fire. You were blameless in all you did from the day you were created until the day evil was found in you. Your rich commerce led you to violence, and you sinned. So I banished you in disgrace from the mountain of God. I expelled you, O mighty guardian, from your place among the stones of fire. Your heart was filled with pride because of all your beauty. Your wisdom was corrupted by your love of splendor. So I threw you to the ground and exposed you to the curious gaze of kings.*
>
> – Ezekiel 28:12–17

Lucifer believed he was better than God and deserved His throne, so he rallied a third of the angels to turn against God. They were all cast out of heaven and out of God's presence as fast as a bolt of lightning.

> *How you are fallen from heaven, O shining star, son of the morning! You have been thrown down to the earth, you who destroyed the nations of the world. For you said to yourself, "I will ascend to heaven and set my throne above God's stars. I will preside on the mountain of the gods far away in the north. I will climb to the highest heavens and be like the Most High." In-*

> *stead, you will be brought down to the place of the dead, down to its lowest depths.*
>
> – Isaiah 14:12–15

Outside the presence of God is darkness and hopelessness. Lucifer became known as Satan. In his rage and anger against God, Satan is determined to take as many people to hell with him as possible.

> *Stay alert! Watch out for your great enemy, the devil. He prowls around like a roaring lion, looking for someone to devour.*
>
> – 1 Peter 5:8

> *Put on all of God's armor so that you will be able to stand firm against all strategies of the devil. For we are not fighting against flesh-and-blood enemies, but against evil rulers and authorities of the unseen world, against mighty powers in this dark world, and against evil spirits in the heavenly places.*
>
> – Ephesians 6:11–12

WHO AM I?

Now that you've been introduced to God and the enemy of your soul, you might be wondering where you fit into the picture. If you have not experienced life-changing salvation and the hope that comes through a relationship with Jesus Christ, my heart aches deeply for you. I can only imagine how difficult grief and loss has been for you without the hope and peace that comes from knowing God.

I'm telling you right now that God created you with a unique calling and purpose. You are more valuable and precious than you could ever fathom. God sacrificed everything through Jesus because of His love for you. A relationship with God and salvation are yours if you confess with your mouth and believe. Scripture gives this assurance:

> *That if you confess with your mouth Jesus as Lord, and believe in your heart that God raised Him from the dead, you will be saved; for with the heart a person believes, resulting in righteousness, and with the mouth he confesses, resulting in salvation. For the Scripture says, "WHOEVER BELIEVES IN HIM WILL NOT BE PUT TO SHAME." For there is no distinction between Jew and Greek; for the same Lord is Lord of all, abounding in riches for all who call on Him; for "EVERYONE WHO CALLS ON THE NAME OF THE LORD WILL BE SAVED."*
>
> – Romans 10:9–13 NASB2020

If you are ready to trust God with your heart and soul, please pray this prayer:

> Lord Jesus, I know that I have sinned and fallen short. I ask for Your forgiveness. You say in Your word that if I confess that You raised Jesus from the dead and accept Him as my Lord and Savior, I will be saved. I confess right now, out loud, that Jesus died on the cross for my sins and that You raised Him from the dead. He is alive! I accept Jesus as my Lord and Savior. Thank you, Father God, for forgiving me, saving me, and giving me eternal life with You. Amen.

When you embrace the salvation that God made available through His Son, Jesus, you bear the title of "child of God" and all that comes with it. For the child of God, the following attributes are true:

- I am a child of God. (John 1:12-13)
- I am filled with the Holy Spirit. (Galatians 5:22)
- I am an heir. (Galatians 4:5-7)
- I am forgiven. (1 John 2:12, Mark 3:28)
- I am loved. (John 3:16)
- I am equipped. (Ephesians 4:11-12, Ephesians 6:11-18)
- I am anointed. (Psalm 92:10)
- I am wonderfully made. (Psalm 139:14)
- I am anointed. (Psalm 92:10)
- I have the power of Christ in me. (Ephesians 3:20-21)
- I am called. (Ephesians 1:18-21, Ephesians 4:1-3)
- I am chosen. (1 Peter 2:9, 1 Thessalonians 1:4-5)
- I am anointed. (Psalm 92:10)

Grief can be all-consuming and cause us to turn our focus inward. One of the things that makes prayer such a powerful weapon is that it shifts our focus outward and upward where it belongs. In the midst of each loss, I pressed in to hear from God. Nothing else mattered. I needed to hear from my Creator, the One who knows me best. I was reminded that I was not alone. I was reminded that my God loves me and fights for me. In time, I began to feel a fire in my heart start to stir again. Watch out, devil!

Recently, I watched a movie called War Room starring Priscilla Shirer as Elizabeth Jordan. I won't give too much away because I highly recommend that you watch this movie if you haven't already. In War Room, Jordan's marriage is struggling, and an older woman in her community teaches her how powerful prayer can be, especially when you feel powerless. There is an epic scene in which Jordan proclaims the truth of God over herself, her marriage, her family, and her home. She declares the following to the enemy:

> I am so sick of you stealing my joy. But that's about to change too. My joy doesn't come from my friends, it doesn't come from my job, it doesn't even come from my husband. My joy is found in Jesus, and just in case you forgot, He has already defeated you. So go back to hell where you belong and leave my family alone![45]

I mention this movie and scene because there is great power in speaking the truth of God out loud. The truth silences the enemy. In moments of great despair, anxiety, or hopelessness, I may feel trapped and overwhelmed as if the season will never end. We have a very real enemy who loves to jump into the middle of those moments and make them feel even heavier and permanent. However, as children of Almighty God, we are not powerless. We don't have to stand by and take a beating. Because of Jesus, we have direct access to the Father who hears our prayers and even commands the armies of Heaven to fight on our behalf.

> *For He will give His angels orders concerning you, to protect you in all your ways.*
>
> – Psalm 91:11 NASB2020

> *This is the confidence which we have before Him, that, if we ask anything according to His will, He hears us.*
>
> – 1 John 5:14 NASB2020

> *For the eyes of the lord are toward the righteous, and his ears attend to their prayer, but the face of the lord is against evildoers.*
>
> – 1 Peter 3:12 NASB2020

> *And if we know that He hears us in whatever we ask, we know that we have the requests which we have asked from Him.*
>
> – 1 John 5:15 NASB2020

> *Then you will call upon Me and come and pray to Me, and I will listen to you. And you will seek Me and find Me when you search for Me with all your heart.*
>
> –Jeremiah 29:12–13 NASB2020

> *Until now you have asked for nothing in My name; ask and you will receive, so that your joy may be made full.*
>
> –John 16:24 NASB2020

I once knew an incredible warrior in the faith whose name was Robert. More than anyone I have known, he taught me how to fight in prayer. Robert experienced everything life could possibly hurl at him from cancer to physical pain to financial hardship, yet his eyes always lit up in the face of opposition or hardship as he declared the goodness of God and told the enemy where to stick it. He would always make it a priority to speak life into everyone he encountered. I have never known anyone like Robert. Even with the struggles he faced, he was always genuinely interested to hear how others were doing. I would share whatever I was wrestling with in the moment, and he would stop me in my tracks and remind me how powerful our God is and tell me that the enemy only has the ground we give him. Robert would pray on the spot, remind the devil that he had no authority, and then speak God's victory over my life. Cancer did ultimately take Robert's life when he was fifty-five years old, but God used every minute while he was with us to claim territory for His Kingdom. That man knew without a doubt who he was in Christ, and he taught me how to fight with the same conviction.

We have been given authority to pray against the schemes of the devil and to speak victory over our lives and circumstances.

GET PRACTICAL

Practice praying right now. Declare the goodness and power of God over your life and circumstances. You are a child of God, and the enemy can't touch you! Tell the enemy and any demonic spirits to flee in Jesus' name. Declare joy and peace in your home. You are a warrior in the faith. Prayer is your weapon. Use it.

WORD OF GOD

> *For the word of God is living and active, and sharper than any two-edged sword, even penetrating as far as the division of soul and spirit, of both joints and marrow, and able to judge the thoughts and intentions of the heart.*
>
> – Hebrews 4:12 NASB2020

For the longest time, I felt completely helpless. I didn't know if I would ever feel freedom or lightness again. I thought heaviness, grief, and anxiety were here to stay. As you know, I frequently vent to God in my journals. One such time, I asked Him why I felt so defeated and powerless. I honestly felt like all my prayers were hitting the ceiling and falling flat on the floor. Why was God allowing the enemy to walk all over me? I was frustrated that God wasn't doing more to rescue me. And then I had this thought, probably prompted by the Holy Spirit: "You are not powerless. You already have everything you need to defeat depression and anxiety." Of course, no additional information was provided. "What do I already have? What?" It took sleeping on it a bit. Then one morning, I woke up at three o'clock, and it hit me! I have the word of God! The Bible describes the word of God as the sword of the Spirit (Ephesians 6:17).

It's the sixth piece of armor mentioned in the armor of God. As Jesus followers, we have weapons that we can use to fight against the enemy and walk as the triumphant children of God we were meant to be. The word of God is powerful enough to create galaxies and the universe, split seas, heal the sick, defeat the enemy, and raise Jesus from the dead. I had access to the word of God the entire time, but I wasn't taking the time to sit and read it and let the truth soak into my heart and soul. By not spending frequent time in the word of God and seeking His direction, I was, in effect, trying to fight the enemy with a toothpick instead of the sword of truth! No wonder I was getting my butt kicked!

My journaling got me in the habit of writing down my thoughts, recognizing lies, and then writing down every possible Scripture verse to combat each lie with God's truth. It made a huge difference for me. Instead of allowing thoughts of anxiety and worry to spin around in my head, I was left thinking about those verses I had written down. The enemy didn't have the power to use his lies against me anymore.

Jesus also demonstrated the power of Scripture when He was tempted by the devil in the desert:

> *Jesus was led by the Holy Spirit to a desert. There He was tempted by the devil. Jesus went without food for forty days and forty nights. After that He was hungry. The devil came tempting Him and said, "If You are the Son of God, tell these stones to be made into bread." But Jesus said, "It is written, 'Man is not to live on bread only. Man is to live by every word that God speaks.'"*
>
> *Then the devil took Jesus up to Jerusalem, the holy city. He had Jesus stand on the highest part of the house of God. The devil said to Him, "If You are the Son of God, throw Yourself down. It is written, 'He has told His angels to look after You. In their hands they will hold You up. Then Your foot will not hit against a stone.'" Jesus said to the devil, "It is written also, 'You must not tempt the Lord your God.'"*
>
> *Again the devil took Jesus to a very high mountain. He had Jesus look at all the nations of the world to see how great they were. He said to Jesus, "I will give You all these nations if You will get down at my feet and worship me." Jesus said to the devil, "Get away, Satan. It is written, 'You must worship the Lord your God. You must obey Him only.'" Then the devil went*

> *away from Jesus. Angels came and cared for Him.*
>
> – Matthew 4:1–11

Cling to His promises and declare the truth of His Word over yourself. Even after I received my promise from God that I would become a mother, I experienced three more miscarriages and received a medical diagnosis of chromosomal translocation giving us a fifty percent chance of having healthy babies on our own. But I clung to that promise and claimed it over and over again even in the midst of our losses. I chose hope over despair, and I claimed God's promise, His word, as my lifeline.

Some days, I have to preach to myself and remind my soul not to give up. I have to speak out in authority that God is still good! I have to speak words of truth over my soul like David did.

> *Let all that I am praise the Lord; with my whole heart, I will praise his holy name. Let all that I am praise the Lord; may I never forget the good things he does for me. He forgives all my sins and heals all my diseases. He redeems me from death and crowns me with love and tender mercies. He fills my life with good things. My youth is renewed like the eagle's!*
>
> – Psalm 103:1–5

GET PRACTICAL

Make spending time in the word of God a daily priority. I'm not talking about being a more dutiful Christian. No! I am talking about spending time in relationship with God. Have a coffee or tea date with the living God who created you and knows you better than anyone else. Don't allow yourself to be defenseless in tough times. Read the word of God. Recite it. Pick up your sword!

WORSHIP

Worship will absolutely feel like the last thing you want to do in the middle of despair, but as soon as songs of worship start to play, the lyrics declare the truth about who God is and what He has done. With worship, God's presence and holiness are invited into your space, and the enemy is forced to leave. Light and darkness cannot coexist. Worry and worship cannot coexist. Worship of the one true God changes our atmosphere in an instant and reminds our spirits that God is in control and can be trusted to keep His promises. His word is the final word. The enemy can take a hike!

> Worship is an act of war against the enemy of our hearts.
> – Holley Gerth[46]

I know what it feels like to wrestle with despair and hopelessness. I can tell you for a fact that in those darkest moments if someone had told me all I had to do was worship, I would have had the following thoughts:

> "You have no idea what I'm going through, or you wouldn't suggest singing right now! Thank you for making me feel like a failure of a Christian for not having chosen a spiritual response to my pain. You must not know what it feels like to suffer. Thanks for your spiritual advice. Let me know when you're actually ready to help."

I certainly didn't feel like worshiping; I had zero motivation to worship. I wanted to hide in the dark and hope that life would forget about me for a while. But I made a choice. I pulled up Spotify on my phone and started playing a worship playlist someone had created. As the music played, the words of the lyrics washed over me. Even if I couldn't bring myself to sing, the lyrics still spoke truth into the room and into my atmosphere.

As I listened to the lyrics, a miraculous thing happened. Every thought of despair, every feeling of hopelessness, every lie of the enemy was silenced in an instant. I felt God's presence, and my anxiety was replaced with peace. I was reminded that I was not alone and that I had value and purpose. It felt like a physical weight was being lifted off me, so I could take a deep breath and exhale. In a matter of moments, my soul was restored.

If you want to see the power of worship in action, read one of my favorite Bible stories as told in the book of Acts written by the Apostle Luke, one of Jesus' disciples:

> *One day as we were going down to the place of prayer, we met a slave girl who had a spirit that enabled her to tell the future. She earned a lot of money for her masters by telling fortunes. She followed Paul and the rest of us, shouting, "These men are servants of the Most High God, and they have come to tell you how to be saved." This went on day after day until Paul got so exasperated that he turned and said to the demon within her, "I command you in the name of Jesus Christ to come out of her." And instantly it left her. Her masters' hopes of wealth were now shattered, so they grabbed Paul and Silas and dragged them before the authorities at the marketplace. "The whole city is in an uproar because of these Jews!" they shouted to the city officials. "They are teaching customs that are illegal for us Romans to practice."*
>
> *A mob quickly formed against Paul and Silas, and the city officials ordered them stripped and beaten with wooden rods. They were severely beaten, and then they were thrown into prison. The jailer was ordered to make sure they*

didn't escape. So the jailer put them into the inner dungeon and clamped their feet in the stocks. Around midnight Paul and Silas were praying and singing hymns to God, and the other prisoners were listening. Suddenly, there was a massive earthquake, and the prison was shaken to its foundations. All the doors immediately flew open, and the chains of every prisoner fell off! The jailer woke up to see the prison doors wide open. He assumed the prisoners had escaped, so he drew his sword to kill himself. But Paul shouted to him, "Stop! Don't kill yourself! We are all here!" The jailer called for lights and ran to the dungeon and fell down trembling before Paul and Silas. Then he brought them out and asked, "Sirs, what must I do to be saved?" They replied, "Believe in the Lord Jesus and you will be saved, along with everyone in your household." And they shared the word of the Lord with him and with all who lived in his household. Even at that hour of the night, the jailer cared for them and washed their wounds. Then he and everyone in his household were immediately baptized. He brought them into his house and set a meal before them, and he and his entire household rejoiced because they all believed in God.

– Acts 16:16–40 NASB2020

Does this story make you want to jump up and declare "Yes!" or what? Paul and Silas were stripped, severely beaten, and then imprisoned in the inner dungeon with their feet clamped in stocks. They were having a really bad day. Instead of despair, even with the excruciating physical pain they must have been experiencing, they choose to sing hymns and praise God. This is truly remarkable! They choose to worship. I love that the passage notes that the other prisoners were listening. Worship changes our atmosphere, and it's so powerful that it impacts those around us too. In this story, an earthquake happens, and everyone's chains fall off. Worship brings freedom. Paul assures the jailer that no one has escaped, and they share the truth of God with the jailer and his entire family. They all receive salvation.

As children of God, we carry authority to change our atmosphere. The enemy will jump right in the middle of our pain and try to convince us that there is no hope or that things will always be like this. We can't let the enemy dictate the narrative in our heads. We are not defeated. We have hope living inside of us. We may feel overwhelmed, out of control, consumed, anxious, depressed, or stressed out, but we have an incredible secret weapon that the enemy will do everything in his power to keep us from remembering: worship! When we are experiencing deep pain, grief, and loss, the last thing any of us feels like doing is worship, but this is when we have a choice. We can either let the enemy keep whispering his lies of despair, or we can turn on worship music and shut him up!

Worship and worry cannot coexist. Worship realigns our spirits with God.

Worship reminds us of who God is, who we are, and it puts the enemy back in his place. We are not powerless. We are not defeated. Don't let the enemy tell you otherwise.

GET PRACTICAL

Pull up these worship songs on YouTube Music or Spotify right now. Listen to the lyrics and allow your soul to come into agreement and remember how powerful and loving and faithful your God is! Remind the enemy of who is in control.

- "Fear Is Not My Future" by Brandon Lake
- "Getting Started" by Jeremy Camp
- "Even When It Hurts (Praise Song)" by Hillsong UNITED
- "So Will I" by Hillsong UNITED
- "Way Maker" by Leeland
- "Fighting For Me" by Riley Clemmons
- "Another in the Fire" by Hillsong UNITED
- "Great Are You Lord" by All Sons & Daughters
- "I Am No Victim" by Kristine Dimarco
- "All He Says I Am" by Kari Jobe
- "Yes and Amen" by Pat Barrett
- "When You Speak" by Jeremy Camp
- "Paul & Silas (At Midnight)" by Naomi Raine and Chandler Moore

Additional worship playlists are available to you via the QR code in the "Resource Library" at the end of this book.

Lifelines

QUESTIONS TO CONSIDER

You have direct access to the God of the universe through prayer. What do you want to tell Him?

Have you ever considered prayer, Scripture, and worship to be weapons? Why or why not?

How do you think your circumstances or mindset might start to shift with more worship?

SCRIPTURE VERSES

Finally, be strong in the Lord and in the strength of His might. Put on the full armor of God, so that you will be able to stand firm against the schemes of the devil. For our struggle is not against flesh and blood, but against the rulers, against the powers, against the world forces of this darkness, against the spiritual forces of wickedness in the heavenly places. – Ephesians 6:10–12

Then you will call upon Me and come and pray to Me, and I will listen to you. You will look for Me and find Me, when you look for Me with all your heart. –Jeremiah 29:12–13 NASB2020

For the word of God is living and active, and sharper than any two-edged sword, even penetrating as far as the division of soul and spirit, of both joints and marrow, and able to judge the thoughts and intentions of the heart. – Hebrews 4:12 NASB2020

Bless the Lord, O my soul; And all that is within me, bless His holy name! Bless the Lord, O my soul, And forget not all His benefits: Who forgives all your iniquities, Who heals all your diseases, Who redeems your life from destruction, Who crowns you with loving-kindness and tender mercies, Who satisfies your mouth with good things, So that your youth is renewed like the eagle's. – Psalm 103:1–5 NASB2020

For the LORD your God is going with you! He will fight for you against your enemies, and he will give you victory! – Deuteronomy 20:4

WORSHIP SONGS

"Yes and Amen" by Pat Barrett.

"When You Speak" by Jeremy Camp.

"Fighting For Me" by Riley Clemmons.

"Getting Started" by Jeremy Camp.

"We Praise You" by Brandon Lake.

"Communion" by Maverick City Music and Steffany Gretzinger.

"Even When It Hurts (Praise Song)" by Hillsong UNITED.

"So Will I" by Hillsong UNITED.

"Way Maker" by Leeland.

"Another in the Fire" by Hillsong UNITED.

"Great Are You Lord" by All Sons & Daughters.

"Fear Is Not My Future" by Brandon Lake.

"Paul & Silas (At Midnight)" by Naomi Raine and Chandler Moore.

"I Am No Victim" by Kristine Dimarco.

"All He Says I Am" by Kari Jobe.

QUOTES

"When the world beats you down, open up your Bible." - Lysa TerKeurst[47]

"I've read the last page of the Bible, it's all going to turn out alright." - Billy Graham[48]

"Worship isn't something we do out of obligation, but rather in response to who God is and what He has done." - Chris Tomlin[49]

"In the process of being worshiped... God communicates his presence to men." -C. S. Lewis[50]

"Without worship we go about miserable." - A. W. Tozer[51]

"The Lord longs to hear all of our concerns. Any concern too small to be turned into a prayer is too small to be made into a burden." - Corrie ten Boom[52]

BOOKS

Fervent: A Woman's Battle Plan to Serious, Specific and Strategic Prayer by Priscilla Shirer.

MOVIES

War Room demonstrates the power of prayer in seemingly hopeless times.

PRAYER

God, thank You for direct access to You through prayer. You hear each one of us. Your Word silences the lies of the enemy and affirms the truth of who You are and who we are in You. Thank You for the power of worship to realign our spirits with Yours and to change our atmosphere. Please remind us that we're not powerless. Give us the courage to pick up our weapons and fight back when our hope and joy are being threatened. In Jesus' powerful name, Amen.

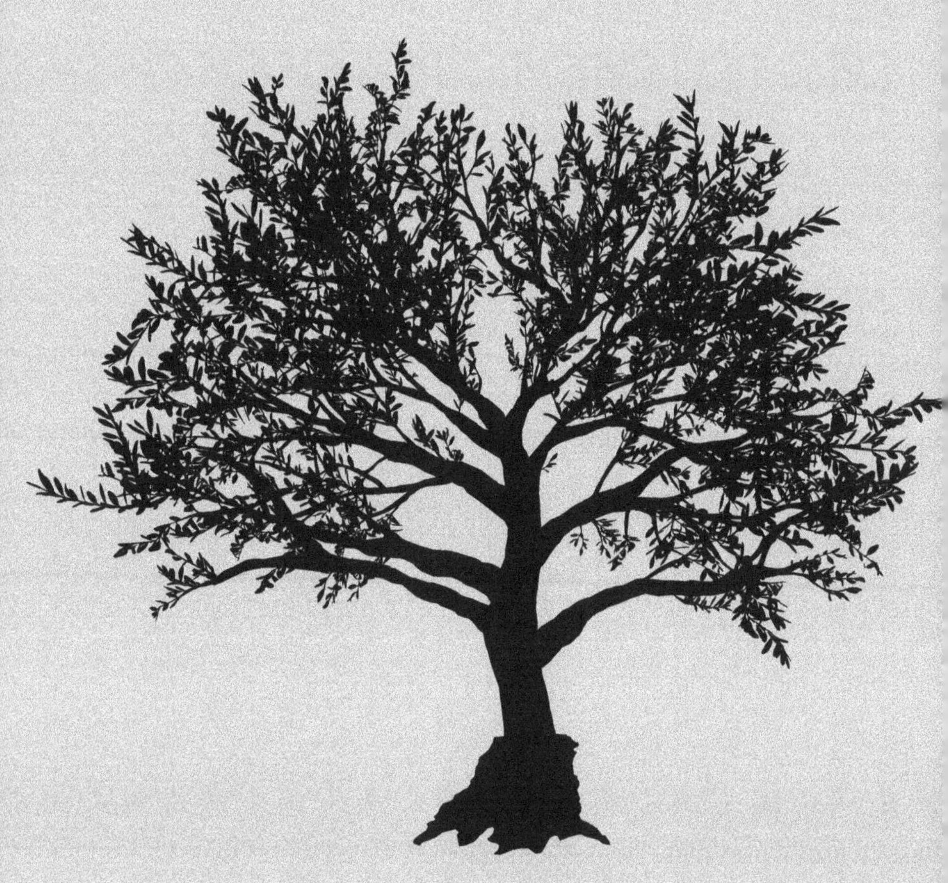

GOD SAID... *I have called you.*

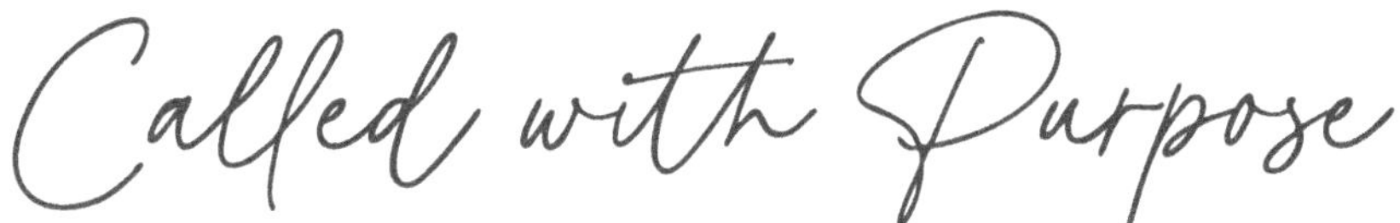

Called with Purpose

Your righteousness, O God, reaches to the highest heavens. You have done such wonderful things. Who can compare with you, O God? You have allowed me to suffer much hardship, but you will restore me to life again and lift me up from the depths of the earth. You will restore me to even greater honor and comfort me once again. – Psalm 71:19–21

I NEVER SAW IT COMING. During my season of darkness, I could barely get out of bed in the morning, let alone imagine a future full of hope and purpose. I would not have believed you if you told me that any good would come out of my losses. I'm grateful that God did not let my story end with loss.

> *And we know that God causes all things to work together for good to those who love God, to those who are called according to His purpose.*
>
> – Romans 8:28 NASB2020

> *Blessed be the God and Father of our Lord Jesus Christ, the Father of mercies and God of all comfort, who comforts us in all our affliction so that we will be able to comfort those who are in any affliction with the comfort with which we ourselves are comforted by God.*
>
> – 2 Corinthians 1:3–4 NASB2020

God began to send friends, strangers, and family members to affirm His purpose and calling for my life. I can be quite stubborn and may have required a neon sign at times. Truthfully, I probably wouldn't have believed a neon sign. I'm glad that God sent so many people to remind me of what I was created and called to do.

The journal entries I share in this section are scattered throughout my entire story from our first miscarriage in 2006 to the present. When looking back through my journals, I was blown away to discover evidence of God speaking into a future I didn't think could be possible. I have set some lines in bold to emphasize when my calling and purpose were being spoken or realized.

> Journal Entry from December 8, 2014:
>
> Things are not always as they seem. Sometimes, it's easy to fall into despair and wonder when the breakthrough will finally happen. I was reading the first page of my most recently completed journal in which I talked about struggling with hope and being afraid of being disappointed. I have to smile because not much has changed in three and a half years. I could have written that entry yesterday. But I also wrote that I choose to trust God with my next steps.
>
> When I bought this journal, I was nervous about the cover being black. To me, black symbolizes death, grief, sadness, and loss. I guess, in a way, it perfectly wraps up this season of my life:
>
> - My stepmom died unexpectedly.
> - We lost our third baby.
> - We struggled financially and signed up for food stamps.
> - I struggled with depression and panic attacks.
> - We received bucket loads of criticism from godly people in our lives.
> - We lost all our possessions (wedding dress, paintings, four years of letters exchanged between Flip and me during our courtship, Christmas decorations, etc.) in a storage unit fire.
>
> On the reverse side, in the midst all the loss and grief:
>
> - I met the Holy Spirit.
> - I received a lot of inner healing.
> - Flip received his calling to open a coffee business.
> - My faith and relationship with God grew.
> - I had a dream about my purpose and calling in life.
> - I ran my first 5K.
> - I lost 40 pounds and two pant sizes.
> - I received the huge blessing of eight boxes of art supplies from a retired artist.
> - We found Fearless LA Church.
> - We were able to tithe every week even without jobs.
> - Our bills got paid somehow.
> - Stocks increased.
> - Flexibility with time permitted me to spend time with God at the harbor.

> God is so good! I am blessed to see all the good that has come through such a season of loss. Thank you, God, for Your faithfulness and never leaving us. In this season of pain and grief, You gave me such a beautiful promise.
>
> *He gives the barren woman a home, so that she becomes a happy mother. Praise the LORD!*
>
> – Psalm 113:9
>
> The one thing I keep reminding myself is that with God, nothing is wasted—no tragedy, no loss, no experience, no hardship—nothing is wasted.
>
> *Everyone will see this miracle and understand that it is the LORD the Holy One of Israel who did it.*
>
> – Isaiah 41:20
>
> *Bring all the tithes into the storehouse so there will be enough food in my Temple. If you do, says the LORD of Heaven's Armies, "I will open the windows of heaven for you. I will pour out a blessing so great you won't have enough room to take it in! Try it! Put me to the test!*
>
> – Malachi 3:10

I feel like the windows of heaven have been opened, and we're awaiting a mighty outpouring of blessing. It may seem crazy or ludicrous to believe or hope in blessing, but I believe that a blessing is right around the corner. This season of grief and loss is coming to a close. We are waking each morning expecting to see God at work on our behalf and in our lives.

We are about to walk, eyes wide open, into the purpose God has called each of us to. It's exciting! At last, my husband will experience his vision of the coffee business come into full reality too. God's promise to me for a home and children will be fulfilled. I will become the person I was intended to be. I will be like Lydia, a merchant of expensive cloth, a worshiper of God, one who attends to the needs of the saints, and is a source of hospitality. I will be like the Proverbs 31 woman providing for my household and bringing honor to my husband. This is what my heart longs for.

I know I am called to "rescue people" from their pit. Although I don't have a clear vision of what that calling looks like yet.

There is a popular worship song that asks the Spirit to lead us beyond the border of our trust. And that's exactly what God did. God began to bring people into my life to speak into my future. I would hear things like, "You're going to speak to many people." "You're a writer."

GO DEEPER

In this section, I reference Gideon's story of reluctance about being called to rescue the people of Israel from the Midianites. Go deeper and read Judges 6:17–27, 36–40, 7:1–8, 9–25 to discover how Gideon progresses from asking God for proof of his calling to timid obedience to overwhelming victory against impossible odds. Along the way, you'll see how Gideon learned to listen and obey God's voice as he overcame fear and confusion and grew from being the least of his tribe to become the mighty warrior God called him to be.

But I felt more like Gideon as I asked: "How can I do these things? I'm weak and broken." Gideon and I are kindred spirits for sure. Look at how he responded to his calling in Judges 6:12–17:

> *The angel of the LORD appeared to Gideon and said, "Mighty hero, the LORD is with you!"*
>
> *"Sir," Gideon replied, "if the LORD is with us, why has all this happened to us? And where are all the miracles our ancestors told us about? Didn't they say, 'The LORD brought us up out of Egypt'? But now the LORD has abandoned us and handed us over to the Midianites."*
> *Then the LORD turned to him and said, "Go with the strength you have, and rescue Israel from the Midianites. I am sending you!"*
>
> *"But Lord," Gideon replied, "how can I rescue Israel? My clan is the weakest in the whole tribe of Manasseh, and I am the least in my entire family!"*
>
> *The LORD said to him, "I will be with you. And you will destroy the Midianites as if you were fighting against one man."*
>
> *Gideon replied, "If you are truly going to help me, show me a sign to prove that it is really the LORD speaking to me.*

Gideon was hiding when the angel of the Lord spoke his identity over him "Mighty hero!" God saw Gideon as the person he was created to be, even though that identity had not been fully realized in Gideon. Gideon pushed back and reminded God that he was part of the weakest tribe.

This is exactly how it was for me when God sent people to speak into my identity and calling. I didn't believe them and then recited to myself all of my shortcomings.

God and I had a chat about my qualifications:

- "I have no idea what I'm doing."
- "Did the Israelites know what they were doing when they entered the Promised Land?" (Joshua 1:1–9)
- "No. They followed Your direction."
- "Did Esther know what she was doing when she became queen?" (Esther 2:1–18)
- "No. She was obedient to follow where You were leading her, and she was alert to opportunities where You could use her in her position."
- "Did Joseph know what was going to happen when his brothers sold him into slavery?" (Genesis 37:18–36)
- "No. He trusted You with his future. He remained alert and looked for opportunities to be obedient to Your leading. He used the gifts and talents You gave him—interpretation of dreams."

God continued to send people into my life to affirm my calling just like He did with Gideon's request for proof of his calling.

> Journal Entry from August 27, 2015:
>
> A breakthrough is around the corner. Last night at UrbanLife (church small group) was amazing. The ladies spoke into my life and future. Nicole texted the following to me on her way home last night:
>
> "So I know while you were speaking, God gave me the name Steffany Gretzinger. She's a worship leader from Bethel and her solo album is really beautiful, really intimate, and raw; her spirit really reminds me of yours. The way you carry yourself. And I know you were talking about how you were trying to find what your calling is, and I know and truly believe that God's calling for your life is greater than you can really imagine. You'll be like a big sister/mom to many. I feel like the trials and tribulations, the deserts, the pits you've hit and gone through are the testimonies that will help others, especially women, find their own identity, and voice, and calling and freedom in God. I really feel like there's a great call of leadership in your life, in the sense that your words will help set people free, break chains and break bondages in their lives. And I asked if you were into the prophetic because I feel like that's one of the areas God will be using you to reach out to others. The visions, words, and melodies God has given you will not go wasted. They will not go in vain. I really feel like they will be used as keys to others so they can unlock their calling and gifts in life. These words will mean so much more to someone else because these words will set them free from something. And this is because I believe that you overflow so much truth, and that's because you're so obedient

> and close to Him. Even just talking to you, I felt like you were so in sync with Him. You have a genuine and powerful spirit that others around you automatically feel how tangible He is because it's so evident in you. You're so loved by God. Like I said, I can really feel His presence around you. There's so much warmth and sweetness when I'm around you, and I know it's because of Him. God bless you and your husband! I will continue interceding for you both. You guys are world-changers. I am so blessed to even have met ya!"

It was incredible to go back and read this journal entry years later and discover how true these words were. I have a voice and a strong calling to point people to God, see chains and bondage broken, and help set people free. I also care very much about unlocking the calling and gifts in others as Nicole spoke over me. It was powerful to read these words and hear Holy Spirit whisper in my ear, "This is who you were created to be."

Like in the story of Gideon, I continued to ask God for more confirmation of my calling, even though He had made it clear to me. God sent me additional people to speak similar words over my life—even from a pastor from Africa who visited our church one Sunday.

> Journal Entry from October 12, 2015:
>
> *A final word: Be strong in the Lord and in His mighty power.*
> – Ephesians 6:10
>
> Good morning, Lord! I praise you! You are so good and so faithful. Thank You for never leaving my side.
>
> I have been asking You to reveal to me who I really am and who I am meant to be. Yesterday, Pastor Jeremy (FearlessLA Church) asked the question, "Who are you when everything is taken away?" If all money, possessions, family, friends, home, etc. are taken away, who am I? What's left? Is God enough for me? Is He my everything? It's a painful question for me to answer because my heart aches and longs for a home and children. But it's a beautiful question because I need to know who I am without those things.
>
> I also met a pastor from Africa at church yesterday. His name is Pastor David. He said that He has preached to 25,000 people and that God has called and anointed him to preach. He asked me if I was a preacher. And I said, "No" and that I'm terrified of public speaking. He said being afraid is good because it allows the Holy Spirit to work. He said he could see me preaching and to be watching for the call within opportunities around me.

It was a wonderful encounter. It left me with a lot to ponder.

God, thank You for revealing who I am in stages. I'm enjoying this adventure. I pray for the courage to walk in obedience to what You have in store for me.

Journal Entry from October 19, 2015:

> *It is better to take refuge in the LORD than to trust in people.*
>
> – Psalm 118:8

> *For I hold you by your right hand—I, the LORD your God. And I say to you, "Don't be afraid. I am here to help you."*
>
> – Isaiah 41:13

God, I want to press into You. I want to go deeper. What is my calling? People around me seem to think I have words to share—a message that will impact others. I don't see myself as a speaker. But I know You see me and all of my potential. You are my everything. I trust You.

Journal Entry from October 23, 2015:

> *The meek also shall increase their joy in the LORD, and the poor among men shall rejoice and rejoice in the Holy One of Israel.*
>
> – Isaiah 29:19 KJV

> *Blessed are the meek, for they will inherit the earth.*
>
> – Matthew 5:5 NIV

My dear friend, Annie, was praying for me and asked God for a word. The word she received was "meek"! She defined it as follows: righteous, humble, teachable, and patient under suffering; long-suffering willing to follow gospel teachings; an attribute of a true disciple.

I want to be known for encouraging others. I want others to feel lifted and lighter after we spend time together. I want to be life-giving. Annie says I have a gift for believing in people.

Journal Entry from October 27, 2015:

God, You call me by name, and You call me "rescuer, advocate, friend." You've called me to join You and rescue others. You've given me a message to share that will break chains. I am a life-giver. I am vitally important. I am deeply loved. I am chosen.

> *But as for me, I will sing about Your power. Each morning I will sing with joy about Your unfailing love. For You have been my refuge, a place of safety when I am in distress.*
>
> – Psalm 59:16

Journal Entry from December 5, 2015:

> *Just as you cannot understand the path of the wind or the mystery of a tiny baby growing in its mother's womb, so you cannot understand the activity of God, who does all things.*
>
> – Ecclesiastes 11:5

I find myself floundering, but the good news is that You know me. I don't need to worry about having all the answers right now. God, I trust You to show me who I am and my calling and purpose in this life. More than anything I want to give life. I would love to create life and have babies and nurture them in everything You desire for them. I want to speak words of affirmation and confidence into others.

I want to dispel words of fear, insecurity, worthlessness either spoken by others or believed in our own thought life. Words are powerful, and the only words that can be trusted come from You, Almighty God. From Your words come life, hope, salvation, that which comes from nothing.

> *His faithful promises are your armor and protection.*
>
> – Psalm 91:4b

> *Let us hold tightly without wavering to the hope we affirm, for God can be trusted to keep His promises.*
>
> – Hebrews 10:23 (emphasis added)

> *Look what happens to mighty warriors who do not trust in God. They trust their wealth instead and grow more and more bold in their wickedness.*
>
> – Psalm 52:7

> *See, God has come to save me. I will trust in him and not be afraid. The LORD GOD is my strength and my song; he has given me victory.*
>
> – Isaiah 12:2

> *Teach those who are rich in this world not to be proud and not to trust in their money, which is so unreliable. Their trust should be in God,*

> *who richly gives us all we need for our enjoyment.*
>
> – 1 Timothy 6:17

God, Your word breathes life into my very being. Impress on my heart truth that I need to hear and deeply believe.

> *For as he thinks within himself, so is he.*
>
> – Proverbs 23:7a NASB2020

God, what is it that I am believing? Help me to see. Please speak truth to my heart. Your words are powerful! I know in my heart that I am a mighty warrior that the enemy fears. Yet I don't know how to embrace my identity.

Journal Entry from January 5, 2016:

Good morning, Lord. Thank You for the rain this morning. God, I am open and ready to receive a word from You. What do you want to do in and through me this year?

The only word that keeps coming to mind is "speak." Speak truth, speak hope, speak courage, speak of God's glory, and speak up. I am afraid of speaking because it invites criticism, offense, and misunderstanding. Words are powerful and should be handled with great care. Words speak life and death. But maybe God has planted a message in me that needs to be shared. Staying silent is worse than facing the risk of criticism. Silence breeds isolation and can also invite misunderstanding. Silence is selfish.

> *But no one can tame the tongue. It is restless and evil, full of deadly poison.*
>
> – James 3:8

> *Gentle words are a tree of life; a deceitful tongue crushes the spirit.*
>
> – Proverbs 15:4

> *The tongue can bring death or life; those who love to talk will reap the consequences.*
>
> – Proverbs 18:21

> *I said to myself, "I will watch what I do and not sin in what I say. I will hold my tongue when the ungodly are around me."*
>
> – Psalm 39:1

> *If you claim to be religious but don't control your tongue, you are fooling*

> *yourself and your religion is worthless.*
>
> –James 1:26
>
> Deliver me, O God, from the fear of being lonely, the need to be accepted, from a life of worldly passions, and the need to be understood.
>
> *The Spirit of the LORD speaks through me; His words are upon my tongue.*
>
> – 2 Samuel 23:2
>
> *Those who control their tongue will have a long life; opening your mouth can ruin everything.*
>
> – Proverbs 13:3
>
> *The mouth of the godly person gives wise advice, but the tongue that deceives will be cut off.*
>
> – Proverbs 10:31
>
> *The tongue of the wise makes knowledge appealing, but the mouth of a fool belches out foolishness.*
>
> – Proverbs 15:2

> ### Journal Entry from August 22, 2017:
>
> Oh, my good friend Nelson also mentioned to me that God wanted him to encourage me to write a book sharing a message of hope. I have felt the nudge to write a book before but didn't take it seriously. I commented that I didn't feel qualified to write, and Nelson pointed to the stack of completed journals on the table. Clearly, I can write. I'm nervous about the journey, but I'm eager to point hurting hearts to hope. God, all I can do is surrender over and over again. Use me. I'm Yours.

> ### Journal Entry from May 25, 2018:
>
> In reading through Mark 6, I find it interesting that the story of Peter walking on water with Jesus is omitted. The gospel of Mark was dictated by Peter, and perhaps he was ashamed to include this part of the story. But it's so significant. I find it easy to be distracted by what I see and forget what God has spoken. Pastor Steven Furtick at Elevation Church agrees; he says, "Anytime I give more focus to what I see than what God spoke, I sink."[53]

It is tempting to leave parts out of our story—to leave the failures out.

If I have learned anything, when God speaks, it happens. To have pastors, friends, family, and even strangers echo the things that God has been speaking to my heart for years is remarkable. If I needed a neon sign, reading these journal entries was it! It's incredible to think that these words were being spoken two years before Jericho was born. In the middle of my brokenness, God was sowing seeds of life into my future.

Additional affirmation of my purpose and calling came through the animated film, Moana, as I watched the movie with my son. At the end of the movie, Moana confronts the lava monster, Teka, while singing these lyrics:

> I have crossed the horizon to find you
> I know your name
> They have stolen the heart from inside you
> But this does not define you
> This is not who you are
> You know who you are[54]

It felt as if God were speaking the same things to my heart, saying, "Your pain does not define you. This is not who you are. I know your name."

I have come to embrace the idea that God can use my brokenness. He restores like no other, and I am called to share my story. Even in this moment, I don't feel qualified, but I can be obedient to the one thing I know I'm supposed to do—that is, to write this book. God will take care of the rest. This book will end up in the hands of those who need it—those who need to be reminded that they are not alone in their pain.

You have a Father God who is more present than you realize. Hope is not gone. Whether you're in the midst of pain right now or starting your healing journey or beginning to come out on the other side with fresh perspective, God is present. He has a word for you. You have a beautiful calling, and your story will change lives. I pray that you will have the courage to look up and trust God with the next step. Press into Him. He will surprise you. There is so much more!

Lifelines

QUESTIONS TO CONSIDER

Have other people ever spoken over you regarding your calling? Do you see a pattern in what they are saying?

Can you see the purpose in your story?

In what ways can you use your pain to comfort others?

SCRIPTURE VERSES

And we know that God causes all things to work together for good to those who love God, to those who are called according to His purpose. – Romans 8:28 NASB2020

Blessed be the God and Father of our Lord Jesus Christ, the Father of mercies and God of all comfort, who comforts us in all our affliction so that we will be able to comfort those who are in any affliction with the comfort with which we ourselves are comforted by God. – 2 Corinthians 1:3–4 NASB2020

Just as you cannot understand the path of the wind or the mystery of a tiny baby growing in its mother's womb, so you cannot understand the activity of God, who does all things. – Ecclesiastes 11:5

Let us hold tightly without wavering to the hope we affirm, for God can be trusted to keep His promises. – Hebrews 10:23 emphasis added

Those who plant in tears will harvest with shouts of joy. They weep as they go to plant their seed, but they sing as they return with the harvest.
– Psalm 126:5–6

WORSHIP SONGS

"You've Always Been" by Unspoken.

"The Story I'll Tell" by Naomi Raine with Maverick City Music.

"Potter and Friend (featuring Jesse Cline)" by Dante Bowe.

"No Fear (Live)" by Kari Jobe.

"Do It Again" by Elevation Worship.

"Voice of God" by Dante Bowe feat. Steffany Gretzinger and Chandler Moore.

"Champion" by Dante Bowe.

"Burn the Ships" by for KING & COUNTRY.

"The Blessing" by Kari Jobe, Cody Carnes.

"Found My Freedom" by I AM THEY.

"Surrounded (Fight My Battles)" by UPPERROOM, Elyssa Smith.

"Defender" by Francesca Battistelli, Steffany Gretzinger.

"I'm Listening" by Chris McClarney, Hollyn.

"God That Saves" by Iron Bell Music.

"See A Victory" by Elevation Worship.

"In Over My Head (Crash Over Me)" by Jenn Johnson, Bethel Music.

SERMONS

"This Is Significant" by Pastor Steven Furtick from Elevation Church: https://sermons.love/steven-furtick/3681-steven-furtick-this-is-significant.html.

"Reclaim Your Calling" by Pastor Craig Groeschel from Life.Church: https://www.life.church/media/called/reclaim-your-calling.

QUOTES

"When we're suffering through hard times, we take God at his Word and believe that he's still in control, with a specific purpose in mind. So we keep going, relying on him. As we keep going, hour to hour, day to day, week to week, we become stronger. Our faith grows, our maturity grows, our trust in God grows. As we get stronger, we believe in God's goodness, more than our circumstances. We learn to believe in God's promises." - Craig Groeschel [55]

"Sometimes when you're in a dark place you think you've been buried, but you've actually been planted." - Christine Caine[56]

"God deliberately chooses imperfect vessels—those who have been wounded, those with physical or emotional limitations. Then he prepares them to serve and sends them with their weakness still in evidence, so that his strength can be made perfect in that weakness." - Christine Caine[57]

BOOKS

Undaunted: Daring to Do What God Has Called You to Do by Christine Caine.

Chase the Lion by Mark Batterson.

Big Jesus: Stories of Faith That Expose the Boxes We Put Him In by Aaron Smith.

PRAYER

Thank you, Jesus, for comforting the brokenhearted. You are so faithful! Thank You for taking my broken pieces, breathing fresh life into my circumstances, and showing me that You had a purpose and plan the whole time. I trust You with my heart, my past, my present, and my future. I'll continue to cling to Your Word as my source. Bring revelation to those who need it right now. Show them that You have never left them—not even for a second. Thank You for healing and for the restoration of hope, joy, and purpose. Only You can change lives and bring beauty from ashes. We claim Your victory today. Thank you for loving us so deeply. In Jesus' name, Amen!

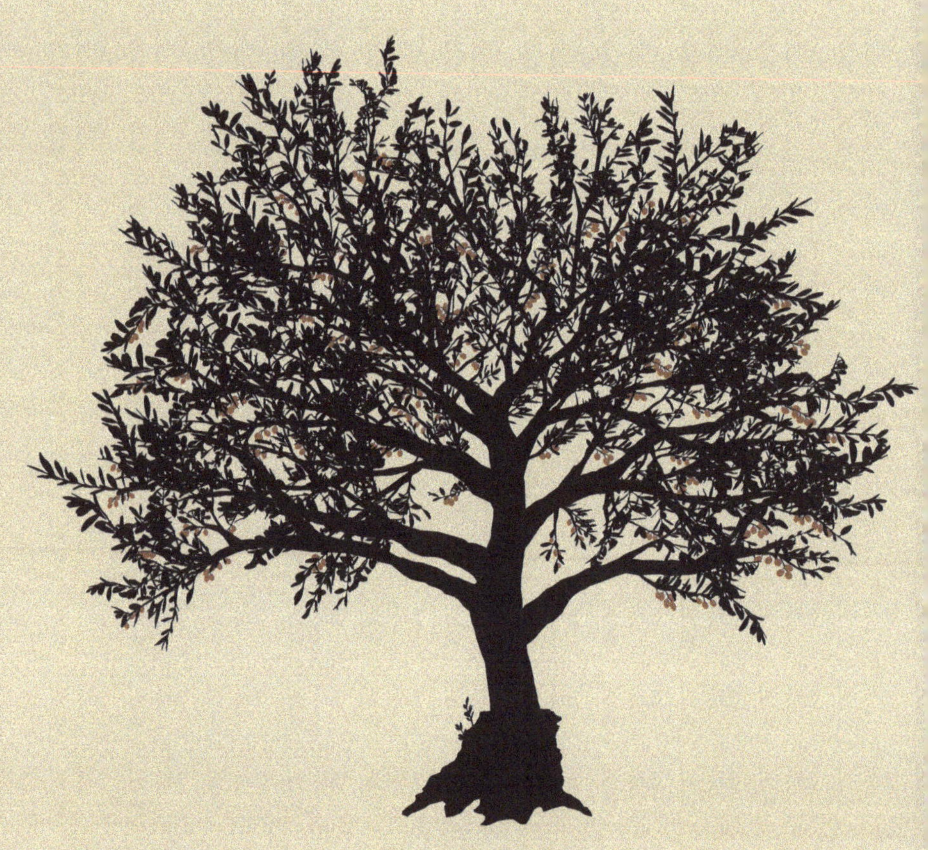

GOD SAID... *immeasurably more!*

So Much More

Now to him who is able to do immeasurably more than all we ask or imagine, according to his power that is at work within us, to him be glory in the church and in Christ Jesus throughout all generations, for ever and ever! Amen. – Ephesians 3:20–21 NIV

GOD GAVE ME A PROMISE IN PSALM 113:9 that He would give me, a barren woman, a home and that I would become a happy mother who would praise the Lord. After six miscarriages, we welcomed Jericho, our miracle, into our lives. Against all odds with a genetic condition, I entered the world of motherhood just as God said that I would.

By the time that Jericho was almost four years old, he had outgrown all his baby clothes, bassinet, infant car seat, accessories, and toys. About that time, very good friends came over to visit. During their stay, they spoke over us that we were going to have more babies of our own. I laughed it off and took it as a compliment or wishful thinking on our behalf. In fact, I even dismissed their words and thought maybe they meant we would adopt or foster in the future, which we were already considering. I resonated with Sarah and Abraham in the Bible when Sarah laughed at the news that she would have a baby. We had not been preventing pregnancy, but after almost four years and one additional miscarriage, we thought we would always be a family of three. After all, God had fulfilled his promise with Jericho.

Then God surprised us. Sure enough—six weeks after our friends' visit, I was pregnant. Having recently donated all Jericho's baby items to moms who needed them, we started over and prepared to welcome our second son, Levi. He was such an unexpected gift. Levi's arrival marked the very first time in fifteen years that I didn't feel broken. God knew that his arrival would bring a deeper level of healing that I didn't even realize I needed. I was able to take a deep breath and embrace my past, be content in my current circumstances, and begin to get excited about the future. I was becoming a happy mother, like my promise in Psalm 113:9 said.

God wasn't about to stop there. He had more in store for us. A year and a half later on my fortieth birthday, we learned that I was pregnant again. We were surprised, especially based on our history. We had no expectations for additional babies, especially with me entering my forties. My doctors didn't let me forget that this was considered a geriatric pregnancy, or that I was of advanced maternal age for having a baby. There's nothing like telling a mama that she's old to make her feel special. Even more than telling me how old I was, they told me how risky it was to have babies this late in life and that my eggs were degraded; therefore, the chance of my baby being stillborn or having a genetic condition was significantly higher.

Had these words been spoken over me when I was pregnant with Jericho, I would have been terrified believing everything they were telling me. With this being my third pregnancy and having witnessed what God can do, their words made me stir with indignation. I immediately prayed a prayer of life and health and protection over my baby. Well-meaning doctors can sometimes instill fear or speak words of death over your unborn baby. If you find yourself in a similar position where people are speaking death over life, surround yourself with life-giving people who will declare, "Your baby is being wonderfully made—God's finest at work." (Psalm 139:13–15) This little one carries a purpose and is meant for great things!" Cling to God and His word. Nothing is impossible for Him. He is the author of life. Keep reciting the truth of the word of God and speak life over your baby. We welcomed our third son, Malachi, into our family, and he is sheer joy. His laugh is the best—it's contagious.

I could never have envisioned how full and beautiful and messy our life is now. With three boys, our home is loud and filled with laughter, pillow forts in the couch, wrestling, dance parties, Legos, trains, and blocks crashing on the floor. I am overwhelmed at the goodness of God. All the noise and chaos represent the volume of blessings in our lives. God fulfilled His promise to me in Psalm 113:9 and so much more than I ever thought possible. Initially, I thought that God would fulfill His promise and that would be it, but I am learning that even now, He's just getting started.

SUCH A TIME AS THIS

God is teaching me that nothing is wasted. He takes pain, heartache, despair, and grief, and He redeems them. He not only restores and heals, but He also rewrites the story into one of triumph. As He says in Jeremiah 29:11, He has a plan of hope and a future for me. It's incredible to see it all unfold and discover that my story was for such a time as this. This story was for you.

It's inspiring to read stories of other people's courage and see how they trusted God against all odds. Esther's story takes trusting God with the outcome to a whole new level:

> *In each and every province where the command and decree of the king came, there was great mourning among the Jews, with fasting, weeping, and mourning rites; and many had sackcloth and ashes spread out as a bed.*
>
> *Then Esther's attendants and her eunuchs came and informed her, and the queen was seized by great fear. And she sent garments to clothe Mordecai so that he would remove his sackcloth from him, but he did not accept them. Then Esther summoned Hathach from the king's eunuchs, whom the king had appointed to attend her, and ordered him to go to Mordecai to learn what this mourning was and why it was happening. So Hathach went out to Mordecai in the city square, in front of the king's gate. Mordecai told him everything that had happened to him, and the exact amount of money that Haman had promised to pay to the king's treasuries for the elimination of the Jews. He also gave him a copy of the text of the edict which had been issued in Susa for their annihilation, so that he might show Esther and inform her, and to order her to go in to the king to implore his favor and plead with him for her people.*
>
> *So Hathach came back and reported Mordecai's words to Esther. Then Esther spoke to Hathach and ordered him to reply to Mordecai: "All the king's servants and the people of the king's provinces know that for any man or woman who comes to the king in the inner courtyard, who is not summoned, he has only one law, that he be put to death, unless the king holds out to him the golden scepter so that he may live. And I have not been summoned to come to the king for these thirty*

GO DEEPER

In this section, I reference Queen Esther's story of fighting fear and courageously imploring the king to save her people from slaughter. Go deeper and read Esther 2:1–23; 4:1–17; 5:1–14; 6:1–14; 7:1–10; and 8:1–17.

- Discover how Esther became queen.
- Unravel an evil plot to massacre the Jews.
- Learn what it takes to silence fear and choose courage.
- Learn about walking in obedience despite all odds and trusting God with the outcome.

days." And they reported Esther's words to Mordecai.

Then Mordecai told them to reply to Esther, "Do not imagine that you in the king's palace can escape any more than all the other Jews. For if you keep silent at this time, liberation and rescue will arise for the Jews from another place, and you and your father's house will perish. And who knows whether you have not attained royalty for such a time as this?"

– Esther 4:3–14 NASB2020

God was strategic in placing Esther in the palace as queen to intervene on behalf of the Jewish people at just the right time. She risked her own life in approaching the king without being summoned. I pray that I have the same courage to walk in obedience to what God is calling me to do. Esther spoke with grace, humility, and wisdom, and God protected her. Justice prevailed, and the Jewish people were saved because of Esther's choice to trust God no matter the outcome.

> Our healing is always for more than just us. It's for all the people on the other side of our obedience.
> – Christine Caine[58]

I have a voice and a strong calling to point people to God, see chains and bondage broken, and help set people free. I also care very much about unlocking the calling and gifts in others. I want to speak words of affirmation and confidence into others. I want to dispel words of fear, insecurity, and worthlessness—whether spoken by others or embedded in your own thoughts. Words are powerful, and the only words that can be trusted come from Almighty God. His words bring life, hope, salvation, and that which comes from nothing.

There is much darkness in this life, but we have the light of the world living inside us. (John 9:5, Matthew 5:14) I have confidence in my God. I have seen firsthand what is possible with Him. His presence comforted me through every loss; His words brought me hope. God held my hand through the darkness and walked me out step by step until I was ready to release my burdens and trust Him with a future I couldn't even fathom. I have learned the freedom that comes from forgiveness. I have experienced what it means to rest in Him and to know that I am not powerless. Prayer, Scripture, and worship continue to be my lifelines and weapons to fight back against any lies the enemy throws my way. I can declare victory no matter what happens because I am a child of God.

She is clothed with strength and dignity, and she laughs without fear of the future.

– Proverbs 31:25

The lyrics from Brandon Lake's song, "Don't You Give Up On Me," have been on repeat in my head like an anthem lately. Brandon wrote the song from God's perspective where God is asking us to not give up on Him during our dark times because He has more dreams, more plans, and more blessings in store for us. I'm living proof of that! There is so much more.

I'm completely in awe of the goodness of God. He gave me a promise (Psalm 113:9) in my desperate need for hope, and He fulfilled that promise with the birth of our son, Jericho. And then He tells me, "Child, we're just getting started." Even now after blessing us with three sons, God is still doing more than I ever could have imagined.

God can be trusted with your heart, your story, and your future too. Watch what He can do! One Word can change everything.

> *"For no word from God will ever fail."*
>
> – Luke 1:37 NIV

Thank You, thank You, thank You, Jesus! You continually surprise me with what's next. You are a God who fulfills promises, who redeems, who restores, and who blesses more than I could ever have hoped or imagined. Only You can take the darkness that comes with pain and turn it into victory. I'm blown away by all that You have done and all that is yet to come. Thank You for Your word and for speaking life into my heart, soul, and future. I'm grateful that I get to do life with You. Thank You for taking my story and turning it into one of hope. Allow others to see that You are a big God and that nothing is impossible with You. Only You! In Jesus' name, Amen!

Acknowledgments

Acknowledgments

GOD: I had a dream once in which I could hear loud clanking and hammering. In the dream, I was irritated that I was being disturbed by the noise. I asked You, "What is going on?" Then I looked up and saw scaffolding on the moon. I asked again, "What is happening here?" You smiled and gently said, "I'm building you the moon, so that your eyes won't hurt when I shed light on the dark and painful places." God, thank You for knowing me so well! I had been holding an incredible amount of pain for so long that it literally felt like I might be buried underneath the weight of it if I dared to even breathe for a moment. Thank You for walking me through the process of healing in a gentle way, step by step. I'm grateful for Your presence and showing me who I was made to be.

HUSBAND: To my champion and confidant. I am incredibly grateful that we get to do life together. I have full confidence that God knew what He was doing when He put us together. You push me and stretch me. You see right through what I would consider weaknesses and speak strength and courage over my life and my future. Thank you for your support and love. Thank you for sacrificing your time to allow me to get this story written. I am eager to see where our obedience in Christ takes us.

MOM: I have this memory of you when I was in ninth grade. I was upset about a situation that had happened at school. I didn't know what to do, and I desperately wanted you to give me advice and tell me what my next steps should be. But instead, you encouraged me to pray about it and ask God for direction. At that moment, I was incredibly frustrated. I wasn't confident that I would receive the help I needed from God. But the truth is that you taught me the greatest lesson of my life that day. God does care about what happens to me, and He is quick to answer when I seek Him and ask for help. Thank you for always pointing me back to God. It is because of your influence that I can boldly say that God is my hope and that He can absolutely be trusted to keep His promises. Thank you!

NELSON: Thank you for speaking over me the title of "writer" in the same way God spoke "mighty hero" over Gideon. I was terrified to see how this story might unfold. Thank you for your words of courage and being consistent in reminding me that I was meant for this.

MARILYN: Thank you for your support and encouragement. Your words breathed life into my passions and dreams again. Thank you for seeing value in me that I couldn't see in myself. I consider myself truly blessed to have had such a fierce warrior advocating for me and pushing me to walk courageously as the person God intended.

TO ALL THE FAMILY MEMBERS AND DEAR FRIENDS who have walked through this journey with me: Your prayers, support, encouragement, and love have meant the world to me. You have reminded me time and again that God did not intend for us to go through life alone. Thank you for your words of affirmation and for gently "pushing" me to move forward in writing this book. It has been a true labor of love, and I could not have done it without you.

TO THE BRANDING CO: I am incredibly grateful for your talents, resources, insights, endless patience, and vision. You truly have a gift for telling a person's story through branding. Thank you.

TO LUCID BOOKS: A huge thanks to the entire Lucid Books Team for partnering with me to publish God Said. Your support, guidance, and expertise have meant the world to me. It would not be possible to publish this story without you. Thank you.

Resource Library

Resource Library

Flippin Baby Testimony
Created by Stephanie Elizabeth Scherer

WORSHIP SONGS

The following public playlists are available on YouTube Music and Spotify.

GOD SAID... hope.

1. "God Help Me" by Unbroken from the *God Help Me EP* album.
2. "Even When It Hurts" by Hillson UNITED from the *Empires* album.
3. "You Know Me" by Steffany Gretzinger from *The Loft Sessions* album.
4. "What I Know" by Tricia from the *Radiate* album.
5. "Out of Hiding" by Steffany Gretzinger from *The Undoing* album.
6. "Sails" by Pat Barrett, featuring Steffany Gretzinger & Amanda Cook.
7. "Open up Let the Light In" by Steffany Gretzinger from *The Undoing* album.
8. "Needing You Now" by Meredith Andrews and We Are Messengers from *My Utmost For His Highest* album.
9. "Rescue" by Lauren Daigle from the *Look Up Child* album.
10. "White Flag" by Fearless BND from the *We Are Fearless* album.
11. "I Am No Victim" by Kristene DiMarco from the *Where His Light Was* album.
12. "Breathe" by Jonny Diaz from the *Everything Is Changing* album.
13. "Pieces" by Steffany Gretzinger from the *Have It All (Live)* album.
14. "Letting Go" by Steffany Gretzinger from *The Undoing* album.
15. "Promises (Radio Version)" by Maverick City Music.
16. "Split the Sea" by Hannah Kerr.
17. "Cover The Earth (Live)" by Naomi Raine.
18. "You Set Me Free" by Angie Miller.
19. "Have My Heart" by Maverick City Music from *Maverick City Vol. 3 Part 1* album.
20. "Be Alright (feat. Amanda Cook)" by Dante Bowe from the *Be Alright* album.

21. "I'm Here For You" by Jonathan Traylor from the *I'm Here For You* album.
22. "Take It All Back" by Tauren Wells from the Joy *In The Morning* album.
23. "Just Be Held" by Casting Crowns from the *Thrive* album.
24. "Through It All" by Ryan Stevenson from the *Wildest Dreams* album.
25. "Oh My Soul" by Casting Crowns from *The Very Next Thing* album.
26. "Joy In The Morning" by Tauren Wells from the *Joy In The Morning* album.
27. "Perfect Peace" by Tauren Wells from the *Citizen of Heaven* album.
28. "Break Your Promises" by Jeremy Camp from the *When You Speak* album.
29. "Worthy of My Song (Worthy of It All)" by Phil Wickham from the *Worthy of My Song* album.
30. "I can't Get Away (Live)" from Melissa Helser and Naomi Raine from *The Land I'm Livin' In* (Live) album.

YouTube Music

Spotify

GOD SAID... *trust.*

1. "Lifting Me Up" by Riley Clemmons from the *Church Pew* album.
2. "Breakthrough (Live)" by Chris McClarney.
3. "Faithful God" by I AM THEY from the *Faithful God* album.
4. "Getting Started (Radio Version)" by Jeremy Camp from the *When You Speak* album.
5. "God Will Work It Out" by Israel Houghton, Naomi Raine, and Maverick City Music
6. "Prophecy Your Promise" by Brian and Katie Torwalt from the *Cafe Sessions* album.
7. "Oceans (Where Feet May Fail)" by Hillson UNITED from the *Zion (Deluxe Edition)* album.
8. "It Is Well" by Kristene DiMarco from the *You Make Me Brave (Live)* album.
9. "You Say" by Lauren Daigle from the *Look Up Child* album.
10. "Another in the Fire" by Hillsong UNITED from the *People (Live)* album.
11. "First" by Lauren Daigle from the *How Can It Be* album.
12. "Say the Word" by Hillsong UNITED from the *Empires* album.

13. "Thy Will" by Hillary Scott & The Scott Family from the *Love Remains* album.
14. "Known" by Tauren Wells from the *Hills and Valleys (Deluxe Edition)* album.
15. "Anchor" by Skillet from the *Victorious* album.
16. "Satisfied" by Jordan Feliz from *The River* album.
17. "Don't You Give Up On Me" by Brandon Lake from the *HELP!* album.
18. "All Along" by I AM THEY from the *Faithful God* album.
19. "Paul & Silas (At Midnight)" by Naomi Raine & Chandler Moore.
20. "Jireh (feat. Chandler Moore)" by Elevation Worship from the *Old Church Basement* album.
21. "Never Leave" by Red Rocks Worship.
22. "Voice of God" by Dante Bowe.
23. "I Will Trust" by Red Rocks Worship from the *Things of Heaven* album.
24. "Give It All" by We Are Messengers.
25. "Tell Your Heart to Beat Again (Remix)" by Danny Gokey.
26. "Carry On" by Tauren Wells from the *Citizen of Heaven* album.
27. "Stay Strong" by Danny Gokey.
28. "Faithfully" by TobyMac from the *Life After Death* album.
29. "Gratitude" by Brandon Lake from the *House of Miracles* album.
30. "Sound Mind (Live)" by Melissa Helser from *The Land I'm Livin' In (Live)* album.

YouTube Music

Spotify

GOD SAID... *victory.*

1. "You Are My Champion" by Dante Bowe from the *Champion (Live)* album.
2. "See a Victory" by Elevation Worship from the *See a Victory* album.
3. "God That Saves (feat. Stephen McWhirter)" by Iron Bell Music from the *God That Saves* album.
4. "The Blessing" by Kari Jobe and Cody Carnes from the *Graves Into Gardens (Live)* album.
5. "In Over My Head (Crash Over Me) (Live)" by Jenn Johnson from the *We Will Not Be Shaken (Live)* album.
6. "When You Speak" by Jeremy Camp from the *When You Speak* album.

7. "You've Always Been" by Unspoken from the *Reason* album.
8. "Do it Again" by Elevation Worship from the *There is a Cloud* album.
9. "Found My Freedom" by I AM THEY from the *Faithful God* album.
10. "Great Are You Lord" by All Sons & Daughters.
11. "Fighting For Me" by Riley Clemmons.
12. "The Story I'll Tell" by Naomi Raine with Maverick City Music.
13. "Potter and Friend (featuring Jesse Cline)" by Dante Bowe.
14. "Fear Is Not My Future" by Brandon Lake from the *HELP!* album.
15. "Burn the Ships" by for KING & COUNTRY from the *Burn the Ships* album.
16. "Surrounded (Fight My Battles)" by Elyssa Smith and UPPERROOM from the *To the One* album.
17. "Defender" by Francesca Battistelli and Steffany Gretzinger from the *Own It* album.
18. "All He Says I Am (featuring Kari Jobe)" by Cody Carnes from the *Gateway Worship– Forever* album.
19. "Yes and Amen" by Pat Barrett from the *Housefires III* album.
20. "I'm Listening." by Chris McClarney and Hollyn from the *Breakthrough* album.
21. "Voice of God" by Dante Bowe.
22. "God Problems" by Maverick City Music from the *Mav Way* album.
23. "Right Where You Want me (Ivory Sessions)" by Sarah Reeves from the *Easy Never Needed You* album.
24. "Miracle" by Riley Clemmons from the Miracle album.
25. "God Be The Glory" by We Are Messengers from the *God Be The Glory* album.
26. "Egypt (Live)" by Cory Asbury.
27. "Again and Again" by Red Rocks Worship.
28. "Desert Song (Live in Australia/2009)" by Hillsong UNITED.
29. "Recover" by Micah Tyler
30. "Take It All Back (featuring Davies)" by Tauren Wells

YouTube Music

Spotify

RECOMMENDED READING LIST

1. *Big Jesus: Stories of Faith Expose the Boxes We Put Him In* by Aaron Smith.
2. *Chase the Lion* by Mark Batterson.
3. *Coming Clean* by Seth Haines.
4. *Crash the Chatterbo*x by Steven Furtick.
5. *Crushing: God Turns Pressure into Power* by T. D. Jakes.
6. *Daring Greatly: How the Courage to Be Vulnerable Transforms the Way We Live, Love, Parent, and Lead* by Brené Brown.
7. *Fervent: A Woman's Battle Plan to Serious, Specific and Strategic Prayer* by Priscilla Shirer.
8. *Fiercehearted* by Holley Gerth.
9. *Get Out of That Pit* by Beth Moore.
10. *Hope in the Dark* by Craig Groeschel.
11. *It's Not Supposed to Be This Way* by Lysa Terkeurst.
12. *Strong, Brave, Loved: Empowering Reminders of Who You Really Are* by Holley Gerth.
13. *Undaunted: Daring to do What God has Called You to Do* by Christine Caine.

BIBLE STORIES SHARED IN THIS BOOK

1. Queen Esther called for "such a time as this" (Esther 4:3–14)
2. The Shunammite woman (2 Kings 4:8–37, 8:1–6)
3. David's candid chat with God (Psalm 77:1–12)
4. Hannah pleads for a child (1 Samuel 1:2–2:21)
5. Noah's Ark (Genesis 6:1–9:17)
6. The walls of Jericho fall (Joshua 6:1–5; 8–16, 20)
7. Paul's list of hardships (2 Corinthians 11:23–27)
8. Paul and Silas praise in prison (Acts 16:16–40)
9. Abraham and Sarah have a son in their 90s (Genesis 17:4–21:2)
10. Gideon called "mighty hero" (Judges 6:12–17)

SERMONS AND ONLINE ARTICLES

1. Frozen Oil and Chosen Vessels by Steven Furtick, Elevation Church, https://elevationchurch.org/sermons/frozen-oil-and-chosen-vessels.
2. "The Other Side of the Promise" by Larry Brey, Elevation Church, https://elevationchurch.org/sermons/the-other-side-of-the-promise-larry-brey.

3. "Hope In the Dark: Waiting on God" by Craig Groeschel, Life Church, https://www.life.church/media/hope-in-the-dark/waiting-on-god.
4. "Where Are You, God?" by Craig Groeschel, Life.Church.
5. "The Courage to Let Go of Your Past" by Christine Caine. YouTube Link: https://www.youtube.com/watch?v=NkNLGASZM7k&t=4s.
6. Tony Martin, "Is It Possible To Forgive God?" The Baptist Record, June 28, 2023, https://thebaptistrecord.org/is-it-possible-to-forgive-god.
7. "Who is Lucifer?" by David Jeremiah, https://davidjeremiah.blog/who-is-lucifer.

Notes

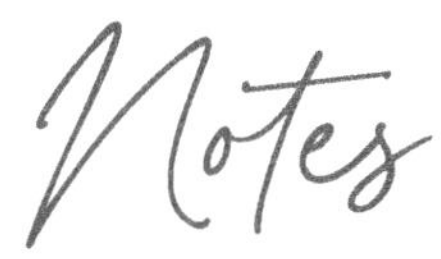

Notes

Preface

[1]Olive Grove Oundle. "What Is So Special About an Olive Tree?" Olive Grove Oundle, accessed August 23, 2023, https://www.olivegroveoundle.co.uk/what-is-so-special-about-an-olive-tree.

PART 1: THE JOURNEY

Hope

[2]Johns Hopkins University, "Dilation and Curettage (D and C)," accessed October 9, 2022, https://www.hopkinsmedicine.org/health/treatment-tests-and-therapies/dilation-and-curettage-d-and-c.

[3]T. D. Jakes, "Crushing: God Turns Pressure into Power," YouVersion Bible App Devotional, accessed January 30, 2020, https://www.bible.com/reading-plans/14679-crushing-god-turns-pressure-into-power.

[4]Nelson Mandela, https://quotefancy.com/nelson-mandela-quotes.

[5]Jakes, "Crushing: God Turns Pressure into Power," YouVersion Bible App devotional.

Faith

[6]Rick Warren, "What Gives Me the Most Hope," Facebook, October 29, 2015. https://www.facebook.com/pastorrickwarren/posts/what-gives-me-the-most-hope-every-day-is-gods-grace-knowing-that-his-grace-is-go/10153665628940903/?paipv=0&eav=AfaZFmVjsVFSkpoepQWKnEgxc55XLGnD7b1x76Wt-FtT6iUp2D8MtlueYESmgCM6sj8w&_rdr.

[7]Steven Furtick, Crash the Chatterbox: Hearing God's Voice Above All Others (Colorado Springs: Multnomah Books, 2014), 66.

[8]Furtick, Crash the Chatterbox, 70.

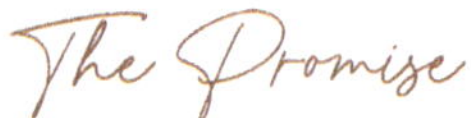

[9]Francis Chan, Christian Central Network, accessed October 9, 2022, https://christiancentral.net/quotes/francis-chan-true-faith-means-holding-nothing-back.

[10]Dwight L. Moody, QuoteFancy, accessed October 9, 2022, https://quotefancy.com/quote/797039/D-L-Moody-God-never-made-a-promise-that-was-too-good-to-be-true.

[11]Charles Spurgeon, Goodreads, accessed October 9, 2022, https://www.goodreads.com/quotes/9044063-the-best-praying-man-is-the-man-who-is-most.

[12]Christine Caine, Undaunted: Daring to Do What God Calls You to Do (Grand Rapids, MI: Zondervan, 2019), 50.

Choosing Trust

[13]Lauren Daigle, "First," How Can It Be album. Centricity Music, 2015.

[14]Brené Brown, QuoteFancy, accessed June 4, 2018, https://quotefancy.com/quote/777660/Bren-Brown-We-cannot-selectively-numb-emotions-when-we-numb-the-painful-emotions-we-also.

[15]Brown, Ibid.

[16]Anne Graham Lotz, QuoteFancy, accessed June 4, 2018, https://quotefancy.com/anne-graham-lotz-quotes.

Daring to Hope

[17]Kimberly Taylor, "Healing Negative Emotions," YouVersion Bible App Devotional, accessed September 6, 2015, https://www.bible.com/reading-plans/1702-healing-negative-emotions/day/4.

[18]Martin Luther King Jr., QuoteFancy, accessed March 17, 2018, https://quotefancy.com/quote/864749/Martin-Luther-King-Jr-Carve-a-tunnel-of-hope-through-the-dark-mountain-of-disappointment.

[19]Craig Groeschel, "Hope In the Dark: Waiting on God," accessed July 30, 2020, https://www.life.church/media/hope-in-the-dark/waiting-on-god.

[20]Jakes, "Crushing: God Turns Pressure Into Power Devotional." YouVer-

sion Bible App. Accessed 20 July 2020. https://www.bible.com/reading-plans/14679-crushing-god-turns-pressure-into-power.

Nowhere but Up

[21]Beth Moore, Get Out of That Pit: Straight Talk about God's Deliverance (Nashville: Thomas Nelson, 2017), 82.

[22]Tim Keller, "How to Deal with Dark Times," (sermon), YouTube.com, uploaded by HTB Church, accessed March 20, 2020, https://youtu.be/ulmaut-baygy.

[23]Furtick, "Walking on Water 101" YouTube, uploaded by Elevation Church, accessed September 10, 2020, https://www.youtube.com/watch?v=_nCn-muIEhzU. Accessed 10 September 2020.

[24]Jakes, Good News Network, accessed on February 22, 2022, https://www.goodnewsnetwork.org/t-d-jakes-quote-about-opposition.

[25]Jakes, AZ Quotes, accessed June 15, 2022, https://www.azquotes.com/quote/1089165.

Jericho

[26]Chris Tomlin, Never Lose Sight Devotional, YouVersion Bible App, accessed January 8, 2017, https://www.bible.com/pt/reading-plans/3161-chris-tomlin-never-lose-sight-devotional/day/7.

[27]The Princess Bride, directed by Rob Reiner, screenplay by William Goldman (1987, Act III Communications, Beverly Hills, CA).

[28]Priscilla Shirer, All Christian Quotes, accessed June 18, 2018, https://www.allchristianquotes.org/quotes/Priscilla_Shirer/3933.

PART 2: THE HEALING

Heart and Mind Preparation

[29]Merriam-Webster.com, s.v. "heal," accessed July 21, 2023, https://www.merriam-webster.com/dictionary/heal.

[30]Merriam-Webster.com, s.v. "health," accessed July 21, 2023, https://www.merriam-webster.com/dictionary/health.

[31]Merriam-Webster.com, s.v. "restore," accessed July 21, 2023, https://www.merriam-webster.com/dictionary/restore.

[32]Merriam-Webster.com, s.v. "renew," accessed July 21, 2023, https://www.merriam-webster.com/dictionary/renew.

[33]Merriam-Webster.com, s.v. "thrive," accessed July 21, 2023, https://www.merriam-webster.com/dictionary/thrive.

[34]Merriam-Webster.com, s.v. " flourish," accessed July 21, 2023, https://www.merriam-webster.com/dictionary/flourish.

[35]Christine Caine, Unashamed: Drop the Baggage, Pick Up Your Freedom, Fulfill Your Destiny. (Grand Rapids, MI: Zondervan, 2018), 113.

The Great Fish

[36]"Fight Or Flight Response," Psychology Tools, accessed July 21, 2023, https://www.psychologytools.com/resource/fight-or-flight-response.

[37]Brené Brown, Brené Brown.com/art, accessed July 21, 2023, https://brene-brown.com/art/24339.

[38]Brown, Brené. Dare to lead: Brave work, tough conversations, whole hearts. (New York, New York: Random House, 2018).

[39]Caine, Unashamed, 125.

Anguish Made Audible

[40]Frozen, directed by Chris Buck and Jennifer Lee (2013, Walt Disney Studios Motion Pictures, Burbank, CA).

[41]Dan Fogelman, (writer), This Is Us, Season 4, episode 18, broadcast on March 24, 2020, 20th Century Fox Television.

[42]Caine, Unshakeable: 365 Devotions for Finding Unwavering Strength in God's Word (Grand Rapids, MI: Zondervan, 2017), 139.

Power in Weakness

[43]Moses, 5 Qualities of the Authentically Strong, A Journey of Faith & Mental Wellness, accessed September 27, 2020, https://brittneyamoses.com/5-qualities-authentically-strong.

Strength in Numbers

[44]Brown, The Gifts of Imperfection: Let Go of Who You Think You're Supposed to Be and Embrace Who You Are (Center City, MN: Hazelden Publishing, 2017), 175.

PART 2: THE HEALING

Stand Firm

[45]War Room, directed by Alex Kendrick (2015, Nashville, TN: Provident Films).

[46]Holley Gerth, Strong, Brave, Loved: Empowering Reminders of Who You Really Are (Grand Rapids, MI: Baker Publishing Group, 2019), 201.

[47]Lysa TerKeurst, QuoteFancy, accessed July 5, 2022, https://quotefancy.com/quote/2316870/Lysa-TerKeurst-When-the-world-beats-you-down-open-up-your-Bible.

[48]Billy Graham, Sermon Quotes, accessed July 5, 2022, https://sermonquotes.com/billy-graham-2/11206-ive-read-last-page-bible-billy-graham.html.

[49]Tomlin, Never Lose Sight Devotional, accessed July 5, 2022, https://www.bible.com/pt/reading-plans/3161-chris-tomlin-never-lose-sight-devotional/day/7.

[50]C. S. Lewis, "Renewing Worship," accessed July 5, 2022, https://www.renewingworshipnc.org/worship-quotes.

[51]A. W. Tozer, QuoteFancy, accessed July 5, 2022, https://quotefancy.com/quote/1447076/Aiden-Wilson-Tozer-Without-worship-we-go-about-miserable.

[52]Corrie ten Boom, "Corrie Ten," accessed July 5, 2022, https://www.quotery.com/authors/corrie-ten-boom.

Called with Purpose

[53]Furtick, "This Is Significant." Elevation Church, https://elevationchurch.org/sermons/this-is-significant, 2018.

[54]Moana, directed by John Musker and Ron Clements (2016, Walt Disney Animation Studios, Burbank, CA).

[55]Groeschel, "Hope in the Dark," devotional, YouVersion Bible App, accessed July 5, 2022, https://www.bible.com/reading-plans/12289-hope-in-the-dark.

[56]Caine, Goodreads, accessed July 5, 2022, https://www.goodreads.com/author/quotes/701214.

[57]Caine, "Undaunted," devotional, YouVersion Bible App, accessed July 5, 2022, https://www.bible.com/reading-plans/14752-undaunted-by-christine-caine/day/7.

So Much More

[58]Caine, Undaunted," devotional, accessed October 1, 2023, https://www.bible.com/reading-plans/14752-undaunted-by-christine-caine/day/7.

www.ingramcontent.com/pod-product-compliance
Lightning Source LLC
LaVergne TN
LVHW052352100826
845147LV00013B/820

* 9 7 8 1 6 3 2 9 6 6 9 2 6 *